YOUR EMOTIONAL TYPE

"*Your Emotional Type* may be the Rosetta Stone we've been waiting for—a code for matching a particular therapy to a particular patient. Micozzi and Jawer . . . have found gold."

LARRY DOSSEY, M.D., AUTHOR OF *HEALING WORDS: THE POWER OF PRAYER AND THE PRACTICE OF MEDICINE* AND *THE POWER OF PREMONITIONS*

"*Your Emotional Type,* securely grounded in scientific research affirming the inseparable unity of mind and body, enables readers to understand how their own personalities may make them prone to a wide variety of health conditions, from chronic fatigue to hypertension, from migraine to fibromyalgia. Most helpfully, the authors guide people to the therapies most appropriate to each personality type. The book is empowering, helping us to become active agents in our healing rather than being simply the recipients of 'cures' from a medical approach that fails to recognize the uniqueness of individuals."

GABOR MATÉ, M.D., AUTHOR OF *WHEN THE BODY SAYS NO: EXPLORING THE STRESS-DISEASE CONNECTION*

YOUR EMOTIONAL TYPE

Key to the Therapies That Will Work for You

Michael A. Jawer and
Marc S. Micozzi, M.D., Ph.D.

Healing Arts Press
Rochester, Vermont • Toronto, Canada

Healing Arts Press
One Park Street
Rochester, Vermont 05767
www.HealingArtsPress.com

Text stock is SFI certified

Healing Arts Press is a division of Inner Traditions International

Note to the reader: *This book is intended as an informational guide. The remedies,
approaches, and techniques described herein are meant to supplement, and not to be a
substitute for, professional medical care or treatment. They should not be used to treat
a serious ailment without prior consultation with a qualified health care professional.*

Library of Congress Cataloging-in-Publication Data
Jawer, Michael A.
   Your emotional type : key to the therapies that will work for you / Michael A.
Jawer and Marc S. Micozzi.
      p. cm.
   Includes bibliographical references and index.
   Summary: "Your emotional type as the means to finding the right treatment for
your chronic illness or pain"—Provided by publisher.
   ISBN 978-1-59477-431-7 (pbk.) — ISBN 978-1-59477-802-5 (e-book)
   1. Medicine, Psychosomatic. 2. Personality — Health aspects. 3. Alternative
medicine. I. Micozzi, Marc S., 1953– II. Title.
   RC49.J39 2011
   616.08—dc23
                                                                    2011030455
Printed and bound in the United States by Lake Book Manufacturing, Inc.
The text stock is SFI certified. The Sustainable Forestry Initiative® program promotes sustainable forest management.

10   9   8   7   6   5   4   3   2

Text design by Virginia Scott Bowman and layout by Jack Nichols
This book was typeset in Garamond Premier Pro with Trajan Pro, Myriad Pro,
Swiss 721 BT and Gill Sans MT Pro as display typefaces

To send correspondence to the authors of this book, mail a first-class letter to the
authors c/o Inner Traditions • Bear & Company, One Park Street, Rochester, VT
05767, and we will forward the communication, or contact the authors directly at
www.emotiongateway.com/pages/furtherinfo/contact.html.

CONTENTS

FOREWORD

People in the United States who are seeking relief from chronic and debilitating health problems, or who want to improve their overall health, are currently investing over $34 billion annually for alternative treatments and approaches that are not offered by mainstream medicine.[1] This expenditure is a dramatic endorsement of complementary and alternative therapies and their effectiveness in addressing a wide variety of physical, emotional, and behavioral problems that seriously interfere with our well-being.

A large number of chronic maladies that plague our modern lives are not the result of germs, faulty genes, or specific traumas. They are developmental in nature, with their roots in our emotional lives. The denial of strong feelings—a process that often takes place completely outside of conscious awareness—can lead to serious disturbances in our bodies' natural processes. The result is a wide array of symptoms and conditions that seriously compromise our ability to enjoy healthy and productive lives. Many of these ills are disappointingly unresponsive to the typical allopathic approaches of pharmaceuticals or surgery.

The vast amount of clinical research devoted to the investigation of alternative health care approaches that have demonstrated their effectiveness is not well known by the general public. Nor do many people know how to assess which kinds of therapy or practice might best serve their needs. *Your Emotional Type* is an extremely useful resource for finding one's way to the kinds of treatments that offer significant—and often dramatic—help to people who suffer from a variety of chronic health problems. These conditions include allergies and asthma, chronic pain and fatigue, depression, fibromyalgia, hypertension, irritable bowel syndrome, migraine headache, phantom pain, rheumatoid arthritis, the skin conditions of eczema and psoriasis, and post-traumatic stress disorder.

Your Emotional Type succinctly reviews the relevant research on complementary and alternative medical approaches that have been proven to alleviate these difficulties. Most of all, it allows you to determine which kind of treatment might be the most useful to *you*, based upon your emotional type, your style of handling strong feelings, and the nature of your health problems. *Your Emotional Type* provides much-needed clarity for those who have not found relief and do not know where to turn.

DEANE JUHAN

Deane Juhan is a practitioner of the Trager Approach and an instructor at the Trager Institute and has developed a series of seminars for all varieties of bodyworkers and therapists, which he presents thoughout the United States, Canada, Europe, and Japan. His previous work as a bodyworker and instructor at Esalen from 1973 to 1990 was his first exposure to the dramatic improvements in a wide variety of conditions that resulted from hands-on work and movement reeducation. His experience leant itself to his books *Job's Body: A Handbook for Bodywork* and *Touched by the Goddess: The Physical, Psychological, and Spiritual Powers of Bodywork.*

Acknowledgments

The authors wish to thank Ernest Hartmann, first and foremost, for supporting our desire to apply his boundaries concept to chronic illness and to complementary and alternative therapies. We also gratefully acknowledge Deane Juhan for his embrace of the book's content and his outstanding foreword; Larry Dossey, Gabor Maté, Ken Pelletier, and Ilene Serlin for their enthusiastic endorsement of the material; and Joel Isaacs of Bodynamic Institute USA for his permission to reprint the bodymap used in figure 1 at the back of the book.

Michael Jawer would like to thank his cherished wife, Bonnie, whose enthusiasm and on-point critiques throughout the book's development were highly welcomed; their kids, Gabrielle and Bradley, who insisted on completing the short-form Boundary Questionnaire themselves; and his parents, Helene and Robert Jawer, for teaching him (though he didn't know it at the time) all about boundaries. Their example, as human beings, parents, and unique (yet compatible) individuals, continues to be an inspiration.

Marc Micozzi would like to acknowledge with gratitude his many colleagues who have reviewed the CAM therapies addressed in this book and whose published work provided a basis for our analysis. He also thanks professors Adi Haramati and Hakima Amri of the CAM program at Georgetown University's School of Medicine, where we lectured on boundaries and administered the short-form Boundary Questionnaire. And thanks to his daughter, Alicia, for completing the questionnaire and making helpful suggestions.

At Inner Traditions/Healing Arts Press we acknowledge Jon Graham, acquisitions editor, and John Hays, director of marketing, for their early recognition of the promise of this project; and Chanc VanWinkle Orzell, project editor. We also wish to thank Marilyn Allen for her constructive questions that helped flesh out the application of boundaries to personality and CAM treatment type.

PREFACE
MARC S. MICOZZI, M.D., PH.D.

It is more important to know what sort of person has a disease than to know what sort of disease a person has.

HIPPOCRATES

There have been many—perhaps too many—books published on alternative medicine and mind-body therapies in the past two decades. But they have all missed an essential element: how do these approaches work for each person as an individual? While physicians and scientists have been preoccupied with the symptoms of illness and how a given treatment works, *Your Emotional Type* matches those treatments with YOUR individual personality type, explaining how they can work for YOU.

Using the personality dimension of boundaries and the spectrum of thick-thin boundary types, described in the opening chapters, *Your Emotional Type* illustrates that different people are sensitive to different stimuli and are susceptible to different ailments. Thick boundary people, for example, are prone to chronic fatigue syndrome and ulcers, whereas thin boundary people are more susceptible to allergies, migraine, and post-traumatic stress disorder. Likewise, not every alternative and complementary therapy will work equally well for each person. Hypnosis is ideal for thin boundary types, for instance, whereas meditation and yoga are better suited to the needs of thick boundary individuals.

The book begins with a crucial yet common-sense declaration: there is no real separation between the brain and the rest of the body, between our heads and our hearts. Every human being is a unified entity, thinking and feeling as one. Our *psyche* (the mental, emotional, and psychological aspects) and our *soma* (the biological, physical, and material aspects) are merely two sides of our commonality. This reality is also why the so-called placebo effect may be so powerful. But beyond the placebo effect, alternative therapies can work wonders for certain chronic conditions . . . as long as they are correctly matched to an individual's boundary type. This breakthrough for a dozen common medical conditions is uniquely addressed in *Your Emotional Type*.

Consumers today are largely overlooked by a health care system that puts each of us into a box based on a disease or disorder, diagnosis, and treatment—what we might call "one size fits all" medicine. This approach works well for the drug companies that develop and dispense medications on a large, industrial scale, designed for a fictitious "standard" person (and designed to maximize profits). But no individual is standard in this way. Everyone reacts to different levels of different stimuli—and each person processes his or her feelings differently. "One size fits all" medicine clearly does not well serve the tens of millions of people today who recognize their own distinct needs by actively pursuing alternative and complementary medical treatments.

Here's a case in point. I was interviewed in 1995 on *Good Morning America* by host Charlie Gibson, when my textbook, *Fundamentals of Complementary and Alternative Medicine* (the first U.S. textbook on the subject, now in its fourth edition), was first published. Cohost Joan Lunden told me she was bothered by shoulder pain from an injury suffered horseback riding. She had tried acupuncture, but it hadn't worked—she had *wanted* it to work, believed that it *would* work, and had many friends for whom it *did* work. If acupuncture were merely a placebo, Ms. Lunden should have derived benefit. The fact that she did not illustrates the real but individualized nature of our physical and emotional well-being—and that even effective alternative medical approaches work better for some people and not as well for others.

For the first time, in *Your Emotional Type,* you will discover, through an easy questionnaire on boundary type, the alternative treatments that will work best for you in alleviating many common conditions for which modern medicine has had no answers.

INTRODUCTION

There is more reason in your body than in your best wisdom.
FRIEDRICH NIETZSCHE, *THUS SPAKE ZARATHUSTRA*

We live in interesting times. In the West, modern medicine has conquered diseases that ravaged previous generations—polio, tuberculosis, syphilis, typhoid fever. Today we are beset by maladies that seem to reflect the prevalence of toxins in our environment and an overload of stress in our lives (such as cancer and heart disease). Modern medicine seems incapable of defeating these ills. Furthermore, people are becoming affected by disorders that were noticed in earlier times but largely ignored in the twentieth century: chronic fatigue syndrome, fibromyalgia, irritable bowel syndrome, and post-traumatic stress disorder. (Notice the word "syndrome" that comes into play. The word *syndrome* indicates that, while the symptoms of a given condition are evident, the cause or connection between them isn't understood. Obviously, then, the condition can't be well treated. These sorts of maladies seem to be increasingly characteristic of modern life.) More and more of us are also made ill by asthma and allergies, while depression casts an ever longer, worrisome shadow.

Perhaps you're among the millions suffering from one or more of these chronic illnesses. Or maybe you have another condition that's problematic, such as migraine headache, hypertension, ulcer, or

1

rheumatoid arthritis. Mainstream medicine has had mixed success (at best) recognizing and treating these various conditions. Moreover, it's "one size fits all" medicine. You as a person get overlooked while your *problems* are evaluated and addressed. Even complementary and alternative medicine (CAM), which is more personalized, raises the questions "What treatment is right for me? And if it works, why does it?"

What is needed is an approach that would bring into sharper focus the factors that lend themselves to various types of chronic illness. Equally valuable would be a way to determine which treatments offer the best chance of success. But where to begin?

Let's start by acknowledging an important but generally overlooked fact: *our feelings have a story to tell.* They alert us to what's going on inside of us, and they draw attention to our reactions to certain events. Like the proverbial tree falling in the woods: if it just misses falling on us—or if it flattens someone we know, or if it flattens *us*—then we'll undoubtedly feel something about it. If it falls somewhere else, though, and we don't hear it or see it, then it's not affecting us and we may feel nothing at all.

Every feeling, then, has a story to tell. It might be a fleeting story, one line ("That ice cream tasted good") or a narrative much more complex ("I can't believe my spouse left me . . ."). Somewhere in that mix, probably closer to the complex side, are the feelings associated with illness. And not just the feelings but often the resulting *symptoms* as well. As you'll gather in this book, many symptoms of chronic illness are clues to the feelings bottled up around them. Symptoms are signposts that, deciphered correctly, tell us something about the personality experiencing them.

That's right—*personality.* Did you think who you are is entirely separate from what you're feeling and what you're going through? Far from it. No one else has your symptoms, your pains and ills. It's you— your body, your self. And, as the Nietzsche quote that started this introduction points out, our bodies have wisdom to dispense if only we're sufficiently tuned in. More wisdom, in the final analysis, than what your doctor tells you or what we, the authors, tell you. Because your lived experiences remain right there, in your body. In many cases, the symptoms you're experiencing can reveal much about the "disharmonies within." (That phrase is borrowed from Chinese medicine, which, like many ancient practices, concerns itself with energies and balance, vitality and flow.[1] See chapter 8.)

Indeed, this book proposes that many chronic conditions have inherent meaning, illustrating nothing less than the characteristic way a person *feels* his or her feelings. Symptoms that you can't shrug off or medicate away, that can't be surgically removed or made to disappear—such chronic conditions are anchored in one's personality, rooted in one's temperament. To be truly understood and unraveled, we must view them in that lived, bodily context.

The word *temperament* comes from the Latin verb *temperare,* "to mix." To "temper" is to adjust or modify something by adding, subtracting, or blending it with something else.[2] Hundreds of years ago, temper was used as a noun by alchemists to refer to a mixture of elements, which led to the present day meaning of temperament as a blend of mental, emotional, and behavioral traits.[3]

This concept of blending continues to hold relevance, because, as we'll see, the displaced *energy of feelings* is implicated in a variety of chronic conditions. That energy is literally *dis*-integrated, with attention called to it through our persistent aches and pains, fatigue, numbness, and so on. By realizing the source and the process that produce these symptoms, we can come home to ourselves, effecting a veritable alchemical transformation.

No, you are not your chronic illness. But it does have personal meaning for you—meaning that can be better disclosed by understanding your *emotional type.* Our term is intended to capture the way different people feel their feelings (or don't). It relates to the brain; it relates to the rest of the body; it relates to your genetic inheritance; and it relates to the way you were raised. Your emotional type indicates how likely you are to be affected by certain chronic conditions. It's a biologically based gauge of personality.

Given the rising incidence of so many chronic conditions—and the difficulty mainstream medicine has in recognizing and treating them—it's not surprising that people are searching for new ways to relieve their suffering. In 2007 (the most recent year for which reliable data are available), more than 38% of American adults spent nearly $34 billion out-of-pocket on complementary and alternative therapies.[4] Equally impressive is the fact that health care workers—especially doctors and nurses—avail themselves of such treatments more often than do the people who consult them.[5] But are all forms of CAM equally beneficial? Are they equally beneficial for *you*?

In *Your Emotional Type,* you'll see how and why your personality type indicates which therapies are best for you. Just as certain people are more susceptible to certain types of chronic illness, those same people will find certain therapeutic approaches more useful. It's ultimately a matter of how much "gets" to you and how you manage intense, energetic feelings. The process is generally automatic and unconscious, and it has been part of you since you were a child. This book will help you unlock that puzzle, shedding new light on your symptoms, your personality, and your style of coping with stressors. *Most of all, you'll have a guide for what to do about it—which CAM treatments are right for you.*

Significant illness has been called a "magnifier of life."[6] It forces us to confront aspects of ourselves we might not otherwise see, surely not to the degree we do when we're in the throes of pain, fatigue, hyperreactivity, or malaise. This means that chronic health conditions offer a unique opportunity to gain insight into who we are. Medical authorities today have just begun to grasp that suffering can yield meaning,[7] but this insight is really nothing new. The Chinese understood it when they stated in the venerable I Ching that "through introspection . . . external obstacles become an occasion for inner enrichment and education."[8]

In this day and age, when information is a mere mouse click away, we have little excuse to simply turn ourselves over to the experts—especially when we have reason to doubt the efficacy of the conventional medical wisdom. *Your Emotional Type* provides an entirely fresh take on the source of your symptoms, why you literally feel the way you do. You'll gain a valuable new framework to augment your health care decisions. Your individuality will be front and center as you gather insight into the ways your personality and your health interact. It's a major step toward true "personalized medicine."

Carl Jung observed that man "can make no progress with himself unless he becomes much better acquainted with his own nature."[9] *Your Emotional Type* will allow you to do just that. By understanding your own style of feeling, you can speed the appropriate form of healing for *you*.

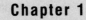

Chapter 1

YOU ARE YOUR BODYMIND

How would you define *personality?* By any definition, it's hugely important to our lives—and even our health. The personality of those closest to us and the interaction with our own personality profoundly affect how we feel and how we get along with family members, bosses, coworkers, neighbors, teachers, classmates, and even the people we encounter casually each day, such as waiters and waitresses, salespeople, or ticket-takers on the local commuter train.

If you're having a bad day, the signals you put out (whether intentional or unintentional) can send other people scurrying. On the other hand, if the person behind the supermarket cash register is having a great day, he or she can lift you out of the doldrums through a megawatt smile, a brief conversation, or just a kindly look. We're social creatures, and highly attuned to each other's moods. But personality itself is something more permanent than mood, more characteristic of one's self. It's the underpinning of whatever the transient signals might be. Think of personality as climate—an overall expectation for a given place over time, regardless of the short-term shifts in temperature, wind, or rain.

The *American Heritage Dictionary* defines *personality* several ways, such as

- the dynamic character, self, or psyche that constitutes and animates the individual;
- the pattern of collective character, behavioral, temperamental, emotional, and mental traits of an individual; and
- the embodiment of distinctive traits of mind and behavior.[1]

Taken together, these definitions reference important concepts: character, mind, psyche, self. The most important aspect, however, might be *embodiment*. We cannot be a self, or have a mind, temperament, or personality, without a body. Surely you've heard the phrase "I'm not feeling myself today." That's said by someone whose experience of him- or herself is a little off, due to how that person is feeling. And a feeling cannot be felt by anyone absent a body.

Now, fast-forward to a news report from the health sciences. It highlights research suggesting that extroverts who have high "dispositional energy"—a sense of innate vigor or active engagement with life—have dramatically lower levels of an immune system chemical known to trigger inflammation. The finding indicates that people who are extroverted and "engaged with life" may be better protected than are other people against inflammatory-related illnesses such as rheumatoid arthritis and stress-related events such as heart attack and stroke. The researchers surmise that a person's engagement level "may reflect a fundamental, biologically based energy reserve, although no one has [yet] explained the biochemistry behind it."[2] This would come as no surprise to traditional Asian medical systems (see chapter 8), in which "vital energy" is considered key to health and disease prevention, causation, and treatment. This vital energy is seen as a fundamental aspect of living beings—it is literally embodied energy.

The researchers behind this particular health story, it should be pointed out, are part of a fast-growing discipline known as psychoneuroimmunology, which studies the interactions between brain and body, the nervous and immune systems, personality and stress, and emotions and health. It's a wide and fertile field of investigation, with fascinating implications for what makes us human.

How energetic we are . . . what we're concerned about . . . what animates or drives us . . . how we feel about ourselves and the life we're leading . . . these are at the crux of personality. It should come as no surprise that our biology is inextricably linked with temperament, health, and, more generally, *how we feel*.

THE ENERGY OF EMOTIONS

That our feelings are dynamic and energetic is easy to demonstrate. Just envision a time you became frustrated or angry and impulsively struck a wall or some piece of furniture. Or consider how drained you can become when worrying about a loved one if that person's health takes a turn for the worse. Take the energy released from crying, by a good belly laugh, or during sexual activity. The amount of energy involved can be immense.

We might picture one of our greatest feelings—joy—as a radiation of happy energy out into the world, and one of our worst feelings—despair—as an inhibition of energy as the individual recedes into him- or herself. That sense of movement is reflected in the word *emotion* itself, which comes from the Latin *emovere,* meaning "to move from" or "to move out of." Such movement is characterized by actual changes in activity within our bodies—changes in the body's chemical profile, in the organs, in the degree of muscle contractions, and in our neural circuitry. In sum, change connotes movement, and movement connotes energy.

While we use calories to measure the intake and expenditure of physical energy, there is no currently accepted "scientific" way to delineate emotional energy. However, an attempt to capture it linguistically has been attempted by many cultures and philosophies (and closely linked to concepts of health and healing). The Hindus call embodied energy *prana;* the Chinese know it as *qi.* Freud found something he termed the libido, and, around the same time as Freud, a French philosopher named Henri Bergson called it *élan vital,* or life force. Whatever we choose to call it, it seems to correlate with the dispositional energy that can protect people from the debilitating effects of stress.

This energy, this *e-motion,* also ties us together. It's rather like a national currency. Our bills and coins go everywhere and are handled by everybody. We may feel flush with cash one day and relatively empty the next, but we *feel* something so long as we're alive. Those feelings are part and parcel of who we are as living beings, as embodied selves who have a personality and the ability to make conscious decisions.

An important qualifier must be added here, namely that personality cannot be reduced to feelings alone. According to a leading personality theorist, Robert Cloninger of Washington University, emotional drives constitute four of seven proposed dimensions of personality. The four are novelty seeking, harm avoidance, reward dependence, and persistence. Together, they make up what Cloninger calls "temperament." The other three dimensions (self-directedness, cooperativeness, and self-transcendence) relate more to conscious abilities and predilections than feelings; these he terms "character." In Cloninger's well-considered framework, character plus temperament add up to personality.[3] Feelings, therefore, can be seen as a foundation of personality—even a driver— but not the entirety in any sense.

THE FAR-FLUNG REACHES OF THE BODYMIND

More than what we think, what we recall, or what we imagine—all of which is considered to be "in our heads"—what ultimately matters is the full body reality of our feelings. The late novelist Milan Kundera put it succinctly: "'I think, therefore I am' is the statement of an intellectual who underrates toothaches."[4]

Indeed, as we go about understanding personality, it's important to take into account a crucial premise of psychoneuroimmunology. Namely, that the brain and the rest of the body are not separate, but integrated and interdependent. And there can be no "mind" without a body. A term that captures this connection is *bodymind,* originated by futurist Ken Dychtwald in his 1977 book of that name.[5]

A helpful analogy is to picture Washington, D.C., and the rest of the country. If you were hosting a foreign visitor and wanted your guest to get to know the United States, you might start with Washington, D.C. (the nation's capital and, in an admittedly limited way, its psyche). But, assuming you had the wherewithal, you'd also want to journey around, taking that person to places like Poughkeepsie, Mobile, Chicago, Bismarck, Salt Lake City, San Francisco (following our analogy, the various parts of the body). We are the "united" states of America—functioning as one country, and a foreigner would not understand us if he or she concentrated solely on Washington, D.C., or on anywhere else.

The bodymind, too, is united. It's the amalgam of brain and body and all internal aspects of us—everything we feel, think, know, intuit, remember, or have forgotten. How does this work? Here's an example. Think for a moment about your most indelible lifetime memory. What was it? Many citizens of a certain age and up would say it was President John F. Kennedy's assassination in 1963. For others, it might be the explosion of the space shuttle *Challenger* in 1986. For still others it could be the time they bungee jumped or skied down a slope they never thought they could. Perhaps it's when you won some major award, received a huge ovation, or heard your beloved say "I do." The more intense the feeling or the more vivid the encounter, the stronger the recollection will be. Experiences that scare, shock, or thrill us are among our most indelible lifetime memories.

Such memories are whole body recollections, relying on connections between the amygdala (a part of the brain that stays on alert for major threats), the vagus nerve (which wanders all the way from the brain to the adrenal glands atop the kidneys), the adrenal glands themselves (which secrete hormones in response to "fight or flight" messages), and the rest of the vital organs and nervous system. The existence of this information loop—combined with the fact that the vagus nerve reaches almost all our internal organs—indicates that our most vibrant memories are encoded not just cognitively in the brain, but viscerally in the body. Furthermore, our vital organs together contain more chemical messengers (neurotransmitters and neuropeptides that are critical of brain activity), than does the brain itself![6] If you've ever had a "gut feeling" or experienced a "heart-ache," you will understand that this is so.

MORE EVIDENCE FOR THE BODYMIND

Science is learning that the supposed line between the brain and the rest of the body is really no line at all. Chemical messengers are crossing it all the time. While researchers speak of the nervous system, or the endocrine system, or the immune system, the concepts are approximate—for study purposes, mainly. Scientists once believed they were separate working systems . . . but no more.

Psychoneuroimmunology is shedding light on the connections. The more that is learned, the more insight is gained on how extensive the overlap really is. *Psychoneuroimmunology*—the term itself—reflects this interface: *psycho* for mind; *neuro* for the neural and endocrine (hormonal) systems; and *immuno* for the immune system.

Take the immune system. In its detection and response to bacteria, viruses, and other foreign invaders, it is crucial, physiologically, to our sense of self.[7] The components of the immune system are located throughout the body: in the thymus (at the base of the neck), the spleen, the lymph nodes (collections of tissue in the armpit, groin, neck, and elsewhere), the bone marrow, the tonsils, and especially the appendix. Immune cells—white blood cells—are sent throughout the body, especially to areas of injury or infection. Their activity produces the familiar inflammatory response as more blood is directed to the affected region and the surrounding tissues swell up.

That the immune system could be influenced by the brain—a truly seminal discovery—was first brought to light in 1975 by psychologist Robert Ader at the University of Rochester. He and his colleagues later advanced the idea that cells are lined with many specific receptors to which only specific molecules can attach themselves. These chemical messengers circulate throughout the body and are the vehicles through which the nervous, endocrine (hormonal), and immune systems communicate.

Such communication goes well beyond the immediate physical connection of neuron to neuron. Within the entire body, various "information substances" are constantly transmitting innumerable messages. Among these substances are peptides: chains of amino acids that are themselves the building blocks of proteins. A given peptide's message is relayed through receptors—sites on the surface of nerve cells through which a given message is transmitted to the cell nucleus. (Peptides associated with the nervous system and brain are labeled neuropeptides.)

FEELING BLUE

Have you ever noticed how one consequence of feeling "blue" for an extended period of time is the greater likelihood of catching a cold or infection? This demonstrates how our state of feeling influences immunity. Stress, too, suppresses immune function through the action of adrenaline and noradrenaline along with other substances (collectively known as corticosteroids) released by the adrenal glands.

Psychoneuroimmunologists have found that such chemical messengers act reciprocally on the brain and the rest of the body. Researcher Candace Pert, then at Georgetown University, noticed a high concentration of peptide receptors "in virtually all locations where information from any of the five senses enters the nervous system." The entire body can thus be characterized as a single sensing and feeling organ: a far-flung, unitary, psychosomatic network.[8]

THE MIND OF THE GUT

Surely you've experienced a "gut feeling" about something from time to time. Perhaps it concerned a relationship that seemed to be going well but somehow gave you pause . . . exchanges at your workplace that didn't seem to add up . . . or a major decision you were on the verge of making but had a nagging doubt about. These feelings don't come out of nowhere but emanate from a very tangible part of our body—the gut.

The gut actually possesses its own self-contained nervous system, known as the enteric nervous system, which can operate in the complete absence of input from the brain or even the spinal cord. It is vast, encompassing more than one hundred million nerve cells in the small intestine alone. When you add the nerve cells of the esophagus, stomach, and large intestine, the result is that the bowel contains *more nerve cells than does the spinal cord*. This makes the enteric nervous system effectively our "second brain."[9]

The enteric nervous system is a vast chemical factory, within which is represented every type of neurotransmitter that can be found in the brain. Think of neurotransmitters as the "words" that nerve cells use to communicate. The lexicon of the brain, then, is fluently spoken by the gut. The stream of messages is so continuous that scientists have begun to refer to sender and receiver as one entity: *the brain-gut axis*.[10]

The term *gut feeling* is no mere figure of speech. Those feelings that bother you, but that you just can't put your figure on, are well worth your time to decipher—and embrace.

HEARTFELT

Other everyday terms about the body are much more than metaphors. How often do you hear phrases like "My heart is full" . . . "She received heart-rending news" . . . "That's a heart-warming story" . . . "What he did was cold hearted" . . . "My heart's just not in it" . . . or "We can embrace that whole heartedly"? The heart is obviously an internal organ with a distinct place in our language, to say nothing of song, literature, and poetry, where it is often "at the heart of" artistic compositions.

For thousands of years, the heart has been regarded as the source of quintessential human qualities—courage, dedication, truth, love. "Take heart," we say to a friend or colleague in need of optimism or faith. Americans place their hands over hearts for the Pledge of Allegiance.

The validity of a statement or idea is recognized when someone says, "In my heart, I know it's true." And where would Valentine's Day be without a heart motif for the chocolates, candies, and greeting cards associated with sweet sentiments?

Scientific evidence is steadily accruing for these associations. Not only have neuropeptide receptors been located in the heart, providing a means for the brain to communicate instantaneously with this most vital of organs, but the heart's atrium area produces a hormone that affects several parts of the brain as well as the pituitary and pineal glands.[11] Studies cited by the Institute of HeartMath (whose express purpose is to advance biomedical research on the heart's energy) suggest that the communication is electromagnetic as well, with the heart's electromagnetic output changing in tandem with the state of bodily feeling.[12] Remarkably, the heart registers by far the strongest electrical and magnetic activity of any organ in the body, including the brain.[13]

Indeed, the heart's projected energy can continue to fill a room long after the people occupying it have left. Equally stunning is the finding that the heart energies of spouses living together can become entrained—that is, their hearts are literally beating together.[14] Further research will quite possibly affirm the traditional view of the heart as the crux of feeling. Given the centrality of feeling to our personal identity, the heart deserves renewed respect as a most critical performer in the "orchestra" that is our bodymind.

A CHANGED VIEW

In general, researchers are discovering that the head is not at all divorced from the heart or the gut, and that our bodily feelings actually underlie and support "mental" activities such as thinking, remembering, and imagining. Feelings are also vital, in the estimation of neuroscientist Antonio Damasio, because they enable us to "mind the body," that is, to recognize (through the heart, the gut, and elsewhere) what is going on inside.[15] Such news is broadcast within us constantly, with moment-by-moment updates.

Clearly, the notion of mind and body as two different things needs to change. Our muscles, our organs, our skin, our nervous system, our endocrine system, our immune system—all are connected, sending cellular and chemical messages to each other continuously and instantaneously. States of health and illness, feeling and mood, reflect the state of the self at any given moment. There's actually no separation between mind and body. It's all one.

This reality is the opposite of what science and philosophy held for centuries. The seventeenth-century French philosopher and scientist René Descartes famously declared, "I think, therefore I am." In light of the recent evidence, though, it would be more accurate to say, "I *feel*, therefore I am."[16]

Seen this way, each of us is psychosomatic. Until recently, that term was often used pejoratively, as in "those symptoms are all in her head—they're psychosomatic." The assumption was made that something either had material reality or was being imagined. *Psychosomatic*, however, literally refers to the whole of who we are: *psyche* (mental, emotional, psychological) and *soma* (molecular, bodily, material). Understood properly, it becomes clear that being psychosomatic is necessary and normal!

Stepping back, there appears to be a genetic angle to bodymind connectivity. An Israeli study done in 2005 provides fascinating insight. Certain people, the researchers found, have an inherited disposition to express their feelings—by dancing. The group of eighty-five performing dancers studied (and their parents) were much more likely than either elite athletes or nondancers and nonathletes to possess variants of two particular genes whose activity has been linked to both spiritual experience and social communication (via the brain chemicals serotonin and vasopressin).[17] The lesson: some people are literally born to dance! Their self, their psyche, their bodymind is geared to communicate to other people how they're feeling. While dance may be the preferred vehicle for some, other people may turn to music, sculpture, or other forms of movement, artistry, and creative expression. All of these, in turn, can benefit health and healing.[18]

LOOKING AHEAD

In the following chapters, you'll see that personality—the "climate" of the way we feel, our distinctively embodied temperament—can be assessed according to a construct called boundaries. This is more than a measure of introversion or extroversion, openness or closed-mindedness, agreeableness or hostility, or any other individual personality trait. Boundaries are a way to assess the characteristic way a person views her- or himself and the way someone operates in the world based on how she or he handles the energy of feelings. To what extent are stimuli "let in" or "kept out"? How are those stimuli processed internally? *Boundaries are a fresh and unique way of appraising human health and functioning.*

In turn, we'll see that a person's boundaries influence not just what is being felt and perceived but also the sensitivities and health conditions to which that person is prone. A person's symptoms, we'll find out, are important but no less so than the entire bodymind—the entire self—who presents them. For indeed, you are your bodymind.

Chapter 2

Our Boundaries, Our Selves

Do you know someone who suffers from migraines? Do you have a friend or family member who's been known to blush at the slightest provocation? Or maybe you know someone affected by a syndrome of some kind: chronic fatigue or chronic pain, irritable bowel, or even post-traumatic stress disorder. Just possibly, you're familiar with someone who seems to internalize the aches and pains presented in the day's headlines or on TV, coming from people halfway around the world. Maybe you yourself are such an empathic person.

If so, you know how the body can throw us for a loop. What you may not fully realize is how feelings invoke these responses within us—and how the symptoms and processes vary depending on the type of person you are. That "type" has to do with boundaries: the characteristic way we recognize what is affecting us, either internally or externally.

For now, consider two scenarios.

First, a therapist is listening to two clients—a wife and her husband—spar over a difficult issue: their sex life. They have a particular dilemma as the wife is a paraplegic (she suffered an accident after they got married). Now, in therapy, she poses the question to her spouse:[1]

"Why don't we have sex any more? I'm still interested." . . . Her husband hung his head, saying little. Then a sudden change: he raised his head, looking directly at his wife and out poured a stream of cruel, cold truth-telling. "I'll tell you why. You think you're normal, but you're not. You won't hear this, but you're disabled. You just lie there, I have to do all the work. Do you know what it's like having sex with a handicapped person? It's not fun, I can tell you." . . . And so on for some considerable time. Then a tearful silence broken eventually by [his wife] in her characteristic upbeat, appealing voice. "Yes, but that's just an excuse, we can try can't we?" The session came to an end and, as the couple left the room, [the therapist] was struck by a powerful and debilitating migraine.

In the counselor's words, "The pain, rage, humiliation, sweetness, desperation, frustration, fear, horror, and heartbreak in the room became too great for me to handle. Taken aback, I identified with everything, it seems: his feelings about living with a paraplegic spouse, her hurt at hearing herself described in this way, and his desperation at her denial. Stunned into silence by the suddenness and the sheer magnitude of this emotional load, I was unable to relieve it. . . . I got a migraine for my troubles."[2]

Scenario two: another therapist feels her clients' concerns manifested though her own aches and pains during therapy. Not only that, she has become aware of "more and more [clients] who feel, in their bodies, the connections between the harming of the planet and their own emotional and physical ailments."[3] An educator and ecologist likewise explains, "The Earth speaks to us through our bodies and psyches. She often cries, and many of us feel her tears and see her pain. I experience it as a force of nature entering me, like light."[4]

Should we take such accounts to be frivolous—or, perhaps, as an indicator of some sort of pathology? Quite the opposite. What people feel has innate meaning and merit. Furthermore, such anecdotes, reported by professionals, shed light on critical personality differences, because not everyone suffers from migraine or feels the pain of the planet. Such differences point up genuine, biological distinctions among individuals. The various ways that people feel relate to the type of "boundary" each person has between him- or herself and the outside world . . . and, indeed, *within* him- or herself.

BOUNDARIES ARE CRITICAL

In the words of psychologist James Hillman, "There is only one core issue for all psychology. *Where is the 'me'?* Where does the 'me' begin? Where does the 'me' stop? Where does the 'other' begin?"[5]

Simply put, our selves require boundaries. From an evolutionary perspective, even the most primitive creatures have a physical boundary (whether skin or another form of membrane) to discriminate "in here" from "out there." The separation allows sensory stimuli to be processed, nutrients to be taken in, and waste products to be discharged. Such a boundary literally defines the individual as a living being.

Over the eons, through the development of nervous systems, some animals became capable of assessing, in a more sophisticated way, what was happening to them and determining what was to be done about it (approach, avoid, chase, etc.). Brain capabilities and functions gradually emerged through this ongoing sensory-based assessment. Indeed, the more advanced a species became, the better it could understand what was happening to it. Not just to receive the incoming stimuli, nor even to "perceive" them, but to link them to their source and be curious about that source.[6] In the case of human beings, this meant to wonder broadly about the world and systematically explore (and exploit) our environment.

As individual selves, we are conscious of our own existence. We notice what is happening to us but we do more—we feel something about it, we think about it, we remember, plan, dream, imagine, create. Because we are *bounded* within our bodies, we are ultimately enabled to have distinct minds and personalities.

HARTMANN'S BOUNDARY SPECTRUM

A fascinating way of looking at personality differences revolves around this very concept. Psychiatrist Ernest Hartmann of Tufts University asserts that each of us can be characterized on a spectrum of boundaries from "thick" to "thin." In his words:

> There are people who strike us as very solid and well organized; they keep everything in its place. They are well defended. They seem rigid, even armored; we sometimes speak of them as "thick-skinned." Such people, in my view, have very thick boundaries. At the other extreme are people who are especially sensitive, open, or vulnerable. In their minds, things are relatively fluid. . . . Such people have particularly thin boundaries. . . . I propose thick and thin boundaries as a broad way of looking at individual differences.[7]

Hartmann first came to his conception in an interesting way. In the 1980s, he was studying people who have nightmares and noticed that they could also readily recall other vivid or colorful dreams even if they didn't qualify as nightmares. These people seemed to him especially "sensitive," "vulnerable," or "imaginative," in contrast with other people, who came across as more "solid," "stoic," or "persevering." He suspected there are real neurobiological differences between thin and thick boundary people, and he developed a questionnaire to gain more insight.

Since the 1980s, at least five thousand people have taken Hartmann's Boundary Questionnaire (BQ), and more than one hundred published papers have referenced it. The scores on the BQ are distributed across the spectrum of boundaries in a bell-shaped curve. Women tend to score significantly thinner than men, and older people tend to score somewhat thicker than younger people.[8]

WHAT WE NOW KNOW

Several other researchers have traversed similar territory over the past two decades. Psychologist Elaine Aron has illuminated various facets of the "highly sensitive person"[9]; Harvard professors Jerome Kagan and Nancy Snidman have studied the differences between "high reactive" and "low reactive" individuals[10]; educator Mary Sheedy Kurcinka has profiled the "spirited child" (one who exhibits high energy as well as pronounced sensitivity)[11]; researchers Sheryl Wilson and Theodore Barber have profiled the "fantasy prone" person[12]; psychologist Sharon Heller has examined factors that make someone "sensory defensive"[13]; and physicians James J. Lynch and Gabor Maté have chronicled "Type C" people, who seem unwilling or unable to acknowledge their feelings.[14]

The accumulated evidence shows that thin boundary people are highly sensitive in a variety of ways and from an early age. They react more strongly than other individuals to sensory stimuli and can become agitated when exposed to bright lights, to loud sounds, or to particular aromas, tastes, or textures. They respond more strongly to physical and emotional pain in themselves as well as in others. They can become stressed or fatigued due to an overload of sensory or emotional input. They're more allergic, and their immune systems are seemingly more reactive. And they were more deeply affected—or recall being more deeply affected—by events during childhood. In a nutshell, they're like walking antennae, whose entire bodies and brains seem primed, in Aron's words, "to notice more in their environment . . . to detect and understand more precisely whatever comes in."[15]

Thick boundary people, on the other hand, are described as stolid, rigid, implacable, or thick skinned. They tend to brush aside emotional upset in favor of simply "handling" the situation and maintaining a calm demeanor. In practice, they suppress or deny strong feelings. They may experience an ongoing sense of ennui, of emptiness and detachment. Experiments show, however, that thick boundary people *don't actually feel their feelings any less*. Bodily indicators (heart rate, blood pressure, blood flow, hand temperature, muscle tension) betray their considerable agitation despite surface claims of being unruffled.[16] This distinction is crucial, as we'll see.

THE BLUSH AND THE MIGRAINE

Let's return to that most commonplace of embarrassments, the blush. When we blush, we are effectively saying that we have feelings we would prefer to deny but cannot. Our reddening face gives us away. (Mark Twain famously stated, "Man is the only animal that blushes. Or needs to.")[17] Such a message not only conveys something to the people we're with but, if we're fortunate, reveals something to ourselves.

There's good evidence that blushing, hypertension (high blood pressure), and migraine headache reflect a similar form of functioning, wherein a thick boundary person—or a thin boundary person who is unconsciously distancing him- or herself from strong feelings—are demonstrating emotional conflict in their bodies. The thick boundary person is constitutionally slow to embrace what he or she is actually feeling, while the thin boundary person may be unaware of the intensity of the feelings he or she is grappling with. (In his book on the subject, neurologist Oliver Sacks observed that migraine is "an oblique expression of feelings which are denied direct or adequate expression.")[18]

Consider the therapist we first met, the one who was struck by a powerful migraine as his spousal clients left the room. Their session had come to involve a devastating exchange of feelings—a combination of "pain, rage, humiliation, sweetness, desperation, frustration, fear, horror, and heartbreak." The therapist recalled that he "identified with everything" and was "stunned into silence by the suddenness and the sheer magnitude of this emotional load." For someone expected to remain objective, what a difficult position to maintain! In his own words, he was ultimately "blindsided, mugged if you like" by a potent mix of feelings that subconsciously penetrated his boundaries.[19]

It's relevant here to note an especially intriguing capacity of the thin boundary person as mentioned by Hartmann. Thin boundary people can generate bona fide physical reactions to a thought, idea, or suggestion. For example, if told to imagine that one is sitting close by a fireplace—or that one is holding an ice cube—a thin boundary person will produce a significantly greater change in skin temperature than someone with thick boundaries.[20] Thin boundary people are not just more highly suggestible, but the evidence shows they are inclined to transmute what they imagine into experiences that are "real as real."

THE FLOW OF FEELING

To better understand this capacity to translate imagination into bodily reality—as well as such phenomena as blushing and migraine—consider the proposition that *feelings are like water*. Picture any given feeling as a flow of clear, cold water, rippling through the body, in continuous motion.

We suggest that this stream of feeling is quicker and more direct in some people (thin boundary types) and slower and less direct in others (thick boundary types). Thus, an especially thin boundary person will seem to be highly sensitive, reactive, even "flighty" because his or her feelings flow quickly through the organism. An especially thick boundary person will, in contrast, appear aloof, imperturbable, even "dull" because his or her feelings proceed more slowly. And while some feelings are wont to register in our awareness, others—the more intensive or threatening kind—can be shunted aside, repressed, or denied.

A blush or a migraine thus reflects the dawning awareness of the feeling or feeling mix. While these experiences may be more characteristic of the thick boundary person (for whom feelings are akin to a foreign language anyway), thin boundary people are not immune from them. A blush, a rash, a migraine, or a bout of chronic pain or fatigue can be said to represent an unconscious assertion of a state of emotional affairs one would rather not consciously acknowledge. The dissonance lurks literally under our skin.

It's interesting to note, in the case of our first therapist, that he no longer suffers from migraines. Why? He's come to recognize the early signs of a headache and realizes that certain feelings must be present. He has literally become more mindful—willing to embrace the reality of furtive emotion—and his headaches have consequently receded.[21]

EXTREME EMPATHY

Let's turn now to our second therapist, the one who literally feels her clients' pain (the Bill Clinton type, you might say). She notices the same process in her clients—that some of them appear to be empathizing with the plight of the earth through their own physical and emotional ills. This degree of empathy is clearly not characteristic of every one of us, but it *is* part and parcel of the markedly thin boundary person.

The process can be seen most clearly in a pair of accounts given by physicians:

- One woman's skin would break out in large hives whenever she was around someone domineering. "Most of her problem involved her mother-in-law, with whom she had a difficult relationship. . . . Whenever she had a memory involving her mother-in-law, she would break out in hives." This included going to the mailbox and finding a letter from her. "And when she talked about her mother-in-law in the psychiatrist's office, [he] would watch the boils form on her skin right in front of him."[22]
- Another woman, with a florid facial rash that had lasted five years, was referred to an immunologist. He found no evidence of allergy, but in reply to his question "What has been the most difficult thing in your life over the last six years?" she promptly answered, "My husband's illness." When asked how it had affected her, she remarked, "Oh, I keep a brave face on it." After she used the same wording again a few minutes later, the immunologist

drew her attention to a possible linkage between her facial rash and the "brave face." A week later, they met again and he provided an opportunity for the patient to discuss her bottled-up feelings. Within another three days, the rash had gone.[23]

That the skin itself can be so sensitive isn't surprising when you consider that a piece of skin the size of a quarter contains more than three million cells, one hundred sweat glands, fifty nerve endings, and three feet of capillaries (small blood vessels). The skin is the largest tissue in the body and is intricately linked to the early development of the immune system, which makes perfect sense given that our skin constitutes the primary physical boundary between "out there" and "in here." In its entirety, our skin contains approximately 640,000 sensory receptors that register heat, cold, pressure, pain, and even electricity.[24]

It's been said that the skin is our body's internal nervous system turned outward—a correct statement since, in the womb, they both develop out of the same surface covering of the embryo.[25] Given this extraordinary sensitivity, we can understand how stress is so closely associated with the skin. Psoriasis, boils, acne, pimples . . . nearly half of skin disorders are estimated to have an emotional component.[26]

The "flow of feeling" mentioned earlier is on vivid display in the cases noted above. Thin boundary people, who have the extraordinary capacity of turning thoughts, memories, images, or suggestions into their own reality, are the ones whose feelings most readily manifest into highly pronounced physical symptoms. Their extreme empathy can cause them to spontaneously become ill, for example, when they see violence on TV or in the movies. It also lends itself to identification with Mother Earth and the pain that some highly thin boundary people feel upon learning about environmental disasters or offenses committed against indigenous peoples still living close to nature.

Recall here Hillman's point about the core issue for all psychology: "Where does the 'me' begin? Where does the 'me' stop? Where does the 'other' begin?" If we do not consider nature the "other"—in the sense that human beings are indisputably part of nature and, even in urban environments, need clean air, clean water, and a modicum of sunshine to live—it's understandable that our ecology would mean something, especially to those of us who have thinner boundaries. Even for those with thicker boundaries, attention to who we are goes hand-in-hand with our surroundings. As poet John Donne wrote in the seventeenth century (and Ernest Hemingway famously repeated in the twentieth): "No man is an island. . . . Do not ask for whom the bell tolls; it tolls for thee."

It's the extreme thin boundary person, though, who most keenly hears the bell toll. In a sense, this personality type is a "bellwether"— a kind of early warning system. Their constitution tends to blur distinctions between "in here" and "out there" that the rest of us take for granted. The ecology—of other people, of animals, of families, of societies, of indigenous peoples, of the planet—lives in them.

EVERYONE IS PSYCHOSOMATIC

As we've seen, human beings literally feel differently based on where we fall along the boundary spectrum. The physical symptoms we present vary also. These boundary differences are thus tangible, verifiable, and lived.

The differences are also bodily. None of us can experience life without a body, so how we think and feel necessarily relates to our sensory experiences, whether current or remembered. Individual consciousness ("self-consciousness") is effectively our perception of how we feel, separate and distinct from other people and whatever else surrounds us.

The various conditions we've surveyed—whether a simple blush, a debilitating migraine, a significant rash, or the pain that comes from too much empathy—point up another lesson that should be self-evident: *we are all psychosomatic.* Our bodies and minds are not only connected, they are one. The symptoms we've assessed are products of whole people, neither residing entirely in their heads nor any other single place.

These symptoms are, in the final analysis, messages from within, emissaries of what we may be feeling but may not yet perceive consciously. They reflect what's known as "the wisdom of the body."

Wherever we may be on the boundary spectrum, each of us is a complex whole, interacting with others who are complex wholes themselves. Whatever we're doing, whatever our interactions, our bodies will be telling a story. The feelings conveyed (or, perhaps, betrayed) are effectively a snapshot of oneself at any given moment. Because the state we're in is conditioned by boundary type, the formulation "our boundaries, our selves" is entirely apt.

The bottom line is this: boundaries offer the most fundamental way of understanding who we are and how we differ, one from another.

PRACTICALLY SPEAKING

The boundaries concept does something else, something vitally useful. It provides a practical frame of reference for the health conditions mentioned in this chapter (migraine, irritable bowel, chronic fatigue syndrome, post-traumatic stress disorder) as well as others that will be addressed later on (hypertension, ulcer, fibromyalgia, and psoriasis, to name a few). Based on where you yourself fall on the boundary spectrum, the types of illness to which you may be susceptible will become clear, *as will the types of therapies that are likely to work better for you.* (Determining your boundary type is easily done—and you can find out in less than ten minutes by taking the short questionnaire in chapter 6.)

Modern medicine is moving toward a model of "personalized medicine" through the knowledge that a person's genetic background inclines him or her toward particular diseases. Not coincidentally, the pharmaceutical industry is aggressively promoting various medications based on how a given person's genes dispose him or her to respond to a particular drug. There's precious little attention, however, given to the basic issues of feeling and personality we've begun to explore in this book.

In the dawning age of personalized medicine, why should health care consumers have to spend thousands of dollars on genetic testing that could violate privacy, jeopardize one's job and insurance, and raise still other concerns? Instead, as we'll see in the next chapter, boundary type can be linked not only to certain chronic conditions but also to alternative and complementary medical approaches that can help. Going down this road, you'll be able to identify and seek out the appropriate remedies *for yourself.* That's true personalized medicine at a fraction of the cost that an exclusive reliance on mainstream medicine now incurs!

Chapter 3

PERSONALITY DIFFERENCES

A Key to Decoding Chronic Illness

Have you ever considered that different people might be prone to different illnesses? We all know that hard-charging Type A people are most likely to succumb to a heart attack—and men are foremost among this group.

But did you know that migraine headache, fibromyalgia, irritable bowel syndrome, and chronic fatigue are predominant among women? Why should this be so? If feelings are fundamental to who we are—and if different people process their feelings differently—there is reason to suppose that individuals would be affected by different conditions based on the *biology* that goes with their characteristic way of feeling.

The whole concept of boundaries captures this important aspect of being human. How you, as an individual, experience what happens to you—how much "gets" to you or how much you shrug off—speaks volumes about the impact your own feelings, and the feelings of others, will have on you. It's nothing more or less than how you experience life!

THE MOST BASIC DIFFERENCE

Let's start with the most fundamental difference between people: gender. The fact is that women are more sensitive, regardless of which sense you look at. Women are accordingly more susceptible to pain, whether physical or emotional.[1]

On the emotional side, one study showed that, for people affected by irritable bowel syndrome, women's brains had greater activity in the limbic region that handles emotion, whereas men had greater activity in their analytical centers.[2]

In general, when under stress the genders react differently. Men are known for the "fight or flight" response, whereas women are more likely to react with "tend and befriend," behavior aimed at calming, understanding, and nurturing in times of trouble. These characteristic reactions probably developed because of the very different social roles of men and women in the evolving human nuclear and extended families of prehistoric times.[3] While men were the hunters and had to make instant life-or-death decisions when faced with harm, women had responsibility for the offspring and would generally have had more time and opportunity to react to an outside threat.[4]

More and more data point to basic biological differences between the sexes. The hippocampus, for example, a brain structure critical to memory, is larger in women, whereas the amygdala, a brain structure that monitors for signals of danger or threat, is larger in men. Furthermore, in women the left side of the amygdala is more active and connected with other brain regions, whereas in men the right side is more active. Because each side of the amygdala channels different neural content, men tend to be more attuned to what's going on *outside* of their body, whereas women are wired to be more aware of what's happening *inside*.[5]

Women also show greater connectivity between the brain's two hemispheres. The rear segment of the corpus callosum—an elongated bundle of nerve fibers that carries information between the brain's two halves—is wider and larger in women than in men.[6] Whether this difference is innately biological or brought about by being treated differently as boys and girls is the subject of debate. But the result is that women tend to have a greater recall of emotional information and a more holistic way of taking into account thoughts, feelings, and the body itself than do men.[7]

These differences can even be seen in the constitution of the brain itself. While men have a significantly greater amount of gray matter (relating to information-processing capacity), women have a larger amount of white matter (representing connections *between* processing centers).[8]

The production of neurotransmitters (the signal-carrying molecules mentioned in chapter 1) differs noticeably, too, with serotonin levels measured at an average 50 percent higher in men.[9] But the relative levels of serotonin may prove to be less important than how, when, and where this chemical actually *works* in the brain.[10]

This point is key because serotonin is known to play a leading role in depression and chronic anxiety, both of which affect women more than men. (The male of the species, on the other hand, experiences alcoholism and impulse control difficulties to a greater degree than women.) By raising serotonin levels indiscriminately to combat depression—which is how Prozac, Zoloft, and other antidepression drugs perform—an essential difference between the sexes is being missed.

We cannot overlook the contribution of sex hormones, either, which obviously differ in the type and amount that circulate through the body. Women's difficulties with mood disorders start to outpace those of men beginning with the onset of puberty, and symptoms can be significantly affected by menstruation as well as pregnancy and the postpartum period.[11] The interaction of estrogen, progesterone, and other hormones with elements of the bodymind's stress-handling system makes for a truly complex web of feelings and inclinations.

Of course, nature does not always trump nurture, and the case will vary depending on the individual woman or man. But you can see why the female of our species—having rapidly gained "equality" in our fast-paced, stress-filled modern culture—might be prone to different sorts of illnesses than the male. Some of that variance might have to do with men being less likely to *report* a given illness—to "suck it up" or "take it like a man." Probably, though, it has a more basic cause, namely that the sexes are configured differently . . . different wiring, different biochemicals, a different sense of one's body, and a different way of processing feelings. All are critically important to the chronic conditions we'll be addressing in order to find the right treatments for *you*.

TWELVE CHRONIC ILLNESSES

Where you fall on the thick-to-thin boundary spectrum is an indicator of which types of illnesses you're prone to. We're not talking *all* illnesses here; just the types that science has shown are most directly related to our thoughts and feelings.[12] These include:

- asthma and allergies
- chronic fatigue syndrome
- depression
- fibromyalgia
- hypertension
- irritable bowel syndrome
- migraine headache
- phantom pain
- post-traumatic stress disorder
- rheumatoid arthritis
- skin conditions such as eczema and psoriasis
- ulcer

These are the twelve—the "Dozen Discomforts"—that this book will primarily address. You'll learn about their correlation with boundary type, the supporting evidence, and then—most importantly—which CAM therapies (CAM is short for complementary and alternative medicine) are most likely to bring you relief.

As we proceed, you'll notice the word *disease* is never used. Instead, this book characterizes each of the Dozen Discomforts as an *illness*, *chronic condition,* or *health condition.* Our operating assumption is that they're each rooted in the bodymind, shaped (albeit unconsciously) by personality and influenced by one's characteristic way of feeling. A *disease,* in contrast, is an illness (even a run-of-the-mill illness, such as a cold) that is *not* primarily conditioned by personality type and the way feelings act within the bodymind. Anyone can catch a cold, and everyone wants to get rid of it. Our bodies try to fight the most serious diseases—such as leukemia, smallpox, AIDS, and cancer—precisely because these are alien and threaten our very survival.

The Dozen Discomforts are different. They are very much *of* us, even if we do not wish them to be. They are somatically and psychically part of our being. They will not be resolved through standard medical interventions (drugs, radiation, surgery, etc.) that treat them as alien. Instead, their meaning—their relationship with oneself—must be understood and drawn out. Through the CAM therapies described later in this book, the aim is for these twelve conditions to be *integrated, transformed,* and *healed,* rather than "cured" in the conventional medical sense.

THERE'S NO SILVER BULLET

Regardless of which condition we look at, most medical researchers want to try to find a single factor, a sole (or at least lead) actor, in a simple cause-and-effect relationship to explain how these conditions work. But that just isn't possible. None of the illnesses we're going to examine is reducible to a single cause—and, therefore, there is no "silver bullet" nor single remedy. These conditions are psychosomatic in the way we defined earlier—they're not merely physical but physical, mental, and emotional *all at the same time.* They take root in the bodymind. Not in the mind and the body as if they're two different things, but in the sum total, the overlap of everything we are.

In this sense, the Dozen Discomforts are very different from cancer, or diabetes, or multiple sclerosis, or hemophilia, or any disease that has a readily identifiable physical basis and originates primarily in the body itself. With these diseases, feelings become involved but mostly after the fact. One's boundary type, or emotional style, does not appear to be the primary reason that one is affected. It's genetics, or diet, or just plain luck. But it's not a matter of an individual's very *being*.

Here is one example of the difference. Chronic fatigue syndrome (CFS) has been around, under different names, since at least 2000 BCE. In ancient China, it was diagnosed as a deficiency of *qi,* or vital energy. (We'll examine the concept of qi in chapter 8.) During the nineteenth century, it was known as *neurasthenia* or, in women, as *hysteria.* Women were always disproportionately affected (*hysteria* is from the Greek word *hysteresis* for "womb"). The cluster of symptoms associated with CFS—disabling tiredness, muscle pain, sleep difficulties, memory problems, headache, depression—was long considered to be a product of the patient's mind. More recently it's been noted, though, that CFS is often preceded by a traumatic event or a viral infection. So it seemed like a breakthrough when an American research team, in 2009, found a retrovirus in the blood of a high proportion of people with CFS.[13] However, two follow-up studies failed to find that same association—so the puzzle remains.[14]

The same story applies to another psychosomatic ailment, ulcers. At first it was generally accepted that stress had a lot do with the development of ulcers. Then, about twenty years ago, Australian researchers produced evidence that a bacterium in the stomach lining, known as *H. pylori,* is responsible. (Ever since medical science developed effective antibiotic cures for germ-caused disease, germs have been the "go to" target for the cause of illness generally.) So, modern medicine dropped the idea of stress and went after killing the bacteria that "causes" ulcers. While it's true that most cases of ulcer—about 90 percent—are associated with *H. pylori,* only about 10 percent of people infected with this bacterium develop ulcers, and another 15 percent of patients don't have it in their stomachs at all. So the "silver bullet" isn't completely convincing. Some other factor—anxiety or stress once again being likely—must be at work, at least with many people.[15]

BACK TO BOUNDARIES

The more that CFS, migraine, fibromyalgia, irritable bowel syndrome, and other conditions are studied, the less they seem explainable by a single cause. At best, they can be lumped into a category that one investigator has labeled "central sensitivity syndrome."[16] The idea is that the nervous systems of people with these conditions literally *amplify* internal or external stimuli—pain, light, sound, smell, touch, whatever. The "whatever" can include emotional prompts like worry, anger, frustration, and trauma. When we talk about such prompts being amplified within the individual, we're talking about boundaries.

From what we know of boundaries, hypersensitivity (another umbrella term) would seem to apply to the thin boundary person. Does that mean *all* of these conditions go with being a thin boundary type? *The answer is no.* As we look at the different illnesses, we'll find that several of them relate to being a thick boundary person. But each of them relates to the way we literally feel our feelings—or don't, as the case may be.

An early proponent of psychoneuroimmunology, George Freeman Solomon, argued that "somatic awareness is akin to psychological insight." He also viewed chronic illness as offering traditional medicine a great challenge: "to arrive at a new integrative theory . . . of disease, of health, of the body, and of the mind/brain."[17] Solomon realized that any chronic condition holds meaning for the affected individual and cannot be understood apart from the self. Given the centrality of feelings to our sense of self and their core role in our personality, an approach such as boundaries offers a fresh, new way to understand these conditions and how they affect people differently.

BROADER THAN BOUNDARIES: THE EXAMPLE OF SKIN AILMENTS

As was noted in chapter 2, the skin is exquisitely sensitive—to the outside world as well as to our own changes in feeling and mood. On the one hand, the skin constitutes a literal boundary between ourselves and others. On the other hand, the skin is our body's internal nervous system turned outward (in the womb, both develop out of the same surface covering of the embryo). Further, the experience of being touched plays a critical role in immune system development in early life.[18]

It shouldn't be surprising, then, that nearly half of all skin disorders may reflect a psychosomatic disturbance.[19] To take a commonplace example, acne—that scourge of adolescence—is definitely worsened by stress. But there are far worse skin conditions, and anyone whose feelings are unrecognized or dissociated may unwittingly contribute to an outbreak.

Psoriasis, a condition in which patches of the skin become inflamed and scaly, is associated—in at least some cases—with rheumatoid arthritis (which, as we'll see, is a thick boundary condition). Eczema, a form of allergy, has been known to occur in conjunction with asthma (which we'll find, along with allergies, is a thin boundary marker). The overall view, then, is that *skin ailments are broader than boundaries.* Anyone with an emotional conflict "under the skin" can conceivably become affected. And anyone who can learn to untangle the conflict can effect a remission. Thin boundary people see the quickest resolution given their higher-than-average ability to identify their feelings and "liberate" the energy that's constrained.

THERAPIES TO FIT THE PERSON

Just as people—and the chronic conditions affecting them—differ according to boundary type, the kind of treatments that work well for one person are bound to differ from the approaches that work for someone else. In general, CAM therapies are well situated to make a difference for people with the Dozen Discomforts, because these approaches are psychosomatic in the literal—and appropriate—sense of the term. They address the emotional/mental ("psyche") as well as the physical ("soma"). They address the whole person, not just the symptoms.

This is especially important when mainstream medicine is stymied by these ailments, with no silver bullets yet found—and none likely to be, either. As one alternative physician puts it (speaking in this case of fibromyalgia), "To try and attack this condition in the classic allopathic sense is like trying to catch the wind in your hand."[20] Even when the condition's functioning is thought to be reasonably well understood—in allergy and asthma, for instance, or migraine, psoriasis, or hypertension—there's more than one facet for medicine to explore. Besides the strictly physical side, there's an emotional side.

This emotional side is the most intriguing aspect of any illness because our feelings energize our entire bodymind and provide a foundation for the self. If we can unravel how a given illness relates to our boundary type, we can better understand what we ourselves are about. The healing that comes with such insight is bound to be durable.

Chapter 4

BOUNDARY SIMILARITIES AND DIFFERENCES

Chronic Fatigue, PTSD, Irritable Bowel, and Fibromyalgia

Words to the wise: *"When we ignore what matters most to us, it will become the matter within us."* This observation, from psychotherapist Paula Reeves, is perfectly in sync with our understanding of the bodymind.[1]

"What matters most" is anything in our lives that holds the most emotional investment—whether we consciously realize it or not. Feelings are a form of energy that is at the core of our selves; if we ignore those feelings or tell them to go away, they won't simply leave without a trace. On the contrary, because they relate to what's highly meaningful, they will hang around. They will bide their time. And they will find a way to become known. As Reeves puts it, they will become the "matter within"—and a potentially unhealthful matter at that.

Through the concept of bodymind, we understand that no complete and utter secrets exist within us. Gut feelings have an inner reality and an inner legitimacy, even though they emanate from our "second brain" down below rather than the upstairs brain with which we're more familiar. A blush, a rash, a migraine, a bout of chronic pain or fatigue: these are all ways that "what matters" within is made manifest. So, too, are conditions such as asthma, depression, hypertension, phantom pain, rheumatoid arthritis, and PTSD.

Feelings (as we gathered in chapter 2) flow like water. In people whose boundaries are thinner, this flow is quicker and more direct. In people who have thicker boundaries, the flow is slower and less direct. Remember, though, that each one of us is psychosomatic—that is, our minds and our bodies are effectively one. Given the differences inherent in boundary type, we can imagine that the stream of feeling will meander different places, and cause different effects, from person to person. In one person, it may pool in a particular locale or ripple over into a tributary. In another person, it may cascade freely. In a third person, the flow may be slowed—dammed up, even.

The characteristic way that someone literally *feels* is bound to influence that person's bodymind symptoms. In many cases, a chronic condition comes to reflect the state of things. If we look closely at these conditions, we will not only see the force of emotion at work, we will see that boundary type can be linked with the given ailment. Thus, *knowing your boundary type is an indicator of the types of chronic illness to which you're susceptible.* For the conditions discussed in this book, your boundary type is just as important, if not more so, than your much-hyped genotype!

Conversely, when we look at these health conditions through the lens of emotion, the ways that they take root (causes) and the ways that they can be resolved (treatments) are illuminated.

The first such illness we'll examine is chronic fatigue syndrome (CFS).

BODY ON THE BRINK

The poet and essayist Susan Griffin has written a remarkable book about her experience with chronic fatigue, entitled, aptly enough, *What Her Body Thought.*[2] Griffin strongly suspects that her early childhood experience—in particular, being treated badly over many years by her alcoholic mother—made her susceptible to CFS. Her suffering, seemingly put out of mind and relegated to the past, reared up out of nowhere in the middle of her eminently successful literary life. Griffin was horrified at what was happening to her and sought to deny the reality of her CFS symptoms. Ultimately, her struggle against the tide was fruitless—because the tide was the very significant "matter within." (The subtitle of Griffin's book, *A Journey into the Shadows,* indicates how she had to make peace with this neglected past.)

To get a sense of how horrendous being afflicted with CFS can be, listen to Griffin's own words:

> In addition to fatigue and general malaise, I had had swollen and painful lymph nodes, terrible headaches, weight loss, mental confusion, memory loss . . . disturbed sleep, night sweats. . . . Odd pricklings, legs, arms, face numb like a foot gone to sleep, only lasting all day. Strange lack of balance, a kind of swimming in the head. A feeling of pressure, as if the brain was swelling. And the inevitable collapse—*fatigue* is too mild a word—that seemed to be coming earlier and earlier each day.[3]

And whereas the idea of bed rest—of peaceful slumber, of comfort between the sheets—sounds appealing to the typical person, for the CFS patient

> the symptoms of illness will more often than not frustrate every attempt you make to get rest. Seriously ill, instead of repose you will find yourself in a pitched battle. You must fight for a few hours of sleep, to gain even a short respite from the pain, to breathe easily or accomplish the simplest bodily chores—brushing your teeth, cleaning your nails, washing your hair.[4]

Not just physical tasks but everyday mental ones become confounding. As Griffin recalls, my memory worsened to the point of absurdity. Trying to think of a practical problem—to remember, for instance, the names of vegetables I wanted friends to purchase when they went shopping for me—seemed beyond my intellectual powers. . . . I experienced the attempt to do so as very tiring, so much so that once when a visiting friend kept asking questions, I burst into tears from the effort to answer her.[5]

In search of an analogy to describe her predicament, Griffin chose the image of "a dilapidated house where every system fails; the same night that a pipe bursts, the electricity short-circuits, and besides the darkness, there is no way to power a pump or even, given that telephones require electricity, call for help. I feel like I lived in such a house, but it was my body . . ." And she characterizes her battle against this unceremonious shutdown as "an elemental struggle for survival," pitting her against something faceless yet insistent, powerful, and unrelenting.[6]

Griffin came to suspect that something was lurking in her past. Something from a nether region of her being, something "still molten" that needed to be turned over, rescued from the dark of neglect or repudiation. She recollected that, during her childhood, "I was often neglected by an alcoholic mother. Too frequently I was left alone, given no dinner, only later to be kept awake by my mother's drunken return." She remembered the fear residing in the then-helpless child, and nights when, in the aftermath of her mother's drinking, she would smell "stale ash and spilled beer . . . and sometimes . . . the faint stench of vomit." These memories brought with them a feeling of acute embarrassment, even shame. Griffin had the sense that bonds of long-ago trust had been irrevocably betrayed, leaving an immense sadness as well as lingering self-recrimination. All of this was still with her, she realized, "experienced even as part of bone, tissue, blood."[7]

DISTANCE FROM FEELINGS

Whereas thin boundary people can be affected any day of the week by a blush, an allergy, a rash, or an ache or pain, thick boundary people are often taken completely unawares by their symptoms. This should not be surprising as the thick boundary person is less than conversant with feelings in general. Thick boundary people tend to "keep on keeping on"; they most often maintain a calm demeanor while denying or distancing themselves from strong feelings. In terms of the Myers-Briggs Type Indicator (MBTI), a popular psychological assessment tool for personality, they score higher on thinking than feeling, higher on sensing than intuition.[8]

The ability of thick boundary people to handle any given situation with a minimum of emotional upset can lead them to take on greater and greater responsibility until they become over-extended personally and professionally. Many people overtaken by CFS—not just Susan Griffin—fit this profile. One of them, a physician, puts it this way (speaking for a group of fellow sufferers): "We [always] felt most comfortable when giving or providing, had difficulty requesting and receiving, and prided ourselves on being available and reliable at all times. Hardworking and even sacrificial, we have been described as driven . . . caretakers . . . with a tendency to overwork and overexert."[9]

It should be emphasized that people who contract CFS are *not* the aggressive, "do it today or you're fired," hard-driving Type A personality. Rather than teeing off on others, they typically blame themselves. Rather than forcing others to shoulder a heavy burden, they will stoically or resolutely carry it alone.

One person who has written about the thick boundary personality (though he refers to it as Type C) is Canadian physician Gabor Maté. He describes people who are used to graciously "taking it" and "taking it"—*until their bodies say no*. Then, abruptly, they find themselves in the position of having to assert "I just can't do it." If they can't stop volunteering or taking on new obligations, they will ultimately have to be cared for themselves.[10]

In Maté's experience, people who are unwilling or unable to express anger, who don't seem to recognize the primacy of their own needs, and who are constantly "doing" are susceptible to a slew of ailments—from rheumatoid arthritis and lupus to multiple sclerosis and amyotrophic lateral sclerosis (ALS, also known as Lou Gehrig's disease). To this catalog should be added chronic fatigue syndrome.

There's one other indication—truly noteworthy—that CFS is associated with the thick boundary personality. A review of twenty-nine studies involving more than one thousand people found that CFS patients are *less amenable to the placebo response* than patients with other illnesses.[11] This result is surprising if one considers CFS to be a "psychosomatic" condition in the traditional sense, namely that its symptoms are all in the person's head. If so symptoms should be able to be reduced through placebos. But only 20 percent of CFS patients improved after receiving placebo treatments, compared with 30 percent of patients with other conditions. We would expect the thin boundary person, who is easily influenced by the power of suggestion, to benefit more readily from placebos. A thick boundary person would not.

TOO MUCH STRESS: THE ORIGINS OF CFS

How does CFS take root? Strong evidence comes from a 2006 study conducted by the Centers for Disease Control (CDC). Four teams of investigators from various fields independently examined data on more than two hundred Americans diagnosed with CFS and concluded that the illness has a verifiable biological basis (as opposed to accusations of patients malingering or being hypochondriacs). Scientists found that people afflicted by CFS tend to have a characteristic set of changes in a dozen genes that help the body respond to stress. One particular combination of gene sequences was found to predict with 75 percent accuracy whether a patient actually had CFS. A correspondence was also found between the severity of an individual's illness and the accumulated stress he or she has faced over a lifetime.[12] These results suggest that the bodymind's stress-handling system is considerably out of kilter for people who suffer from CFS. They are not simply tired or depressed.

Scientifically speaking, the hypothalamic-pituitary-adrenal axis, or HPA axis for short, is a critical part of our stress-activation system. Its operation is influenced by genetics but also by the type and frequency of stressors that one encounters. Thus, the HPA "set point" will differ from person to person. In some people, it's set relatively high; these are the folks who appear calm and collected in almost any circumstance. In other people, the HPA set point is relatively low; they are the "high reactors" who typically appear jumpy or nervous.[13] (Picture Don Knotts as Officer Barney Fife in the 1960s *Andy Griffith* TV show.) The key thing to realize: while nature may predispose some of us to be especially thick (low reacting) or especially thin (high reacting), genetics is not the whole story. The functioning of the HPA axis will change based on environmental influences, too. Early life experiences, especially parental care, can exert a significant effect.[14]

It's noteworthy that one of the CDC researchers found evidence that childhood trauma—especially sexual abuse and physical or emotional neglect—increases the odds of CFS occurring later on in life *six to eight times*.[15] Similarly, a Swedish study determined that high levels of stress—even if occurring decades before one's CFS symptoms—make it two-thirds more likely that a person will have the condition.[16] These remarkable findings indicate that CFS evolves from early and severe stress.

Think of Susan Griffin's upbringing with an often absent, alcoholic mother. Or, picture any child of the thick boundary type, who is naturally somewhat distanced from her or his feelings. Severe, chronic stress *should* engender emotional upset—but this is a bit of a challenge for the thick boundary person. That individual's tendency is to soldier on, to deny the meaningfulness of strong feelings or unconsciously detach from them. Remember, though, from chapter 2 that thick boundary people don't actually feel their feelings any less. Their bodies (through indicators such as heart rate, blood pressure, blood flow, hand temperature, and muscle tension) verify they *are* upset, even if they don't realize it. Consciously, they may have a suspicion that something is amiss because they literally feel numb for a time. They've become *dissociated* from the power of their feelings.

The energy of those feelings, though, doesn't disappear—it goes "underground" within the bodymind. There it remains for many years, stagnant (to use our water analogy). As an adult, the thick boundary person doesn't even realize that the events in childhood were significant or even traumatic emotionally. Yet the buried recollections—and their emotional energy—remain.

THE CFS TRIGGER

In cases of CFS, something eventually happens to throw off the old order. What could it be? Some sort of stimulus—a sight, a smell, a passing remark—flies in under the person's radar. This prompt needn't be very large, but it bears some relation to the original circumstances. The person's natural inclination is, once again, to deny or minimize the validity of what is happening. But the very effort involved in suppressing feelings requires energy! *The individual will become fatigued because the effort needed to keep the long-relegated feelings at bay saps all of his or her resources.* Meanwhile, the person's life is turned staggeringly upside down as the CFS symptoms take hold.

Two well-known researchers into the psychosomatic effects of stress—Ronald Glaser and Janice Kiecolt-Glaser at Ohio State University—have proposed an origin for CFS that approximates the model presented here. Their idea is that increased stress can activate viruses long present in the body but existing under the immune system's activation threshold.[17] Substitute "dissociated energy" for "virus" and "HPA axis" for "immune system" and you have the idea. While we acknowledge that the body's stress reaction to a low-grade infection *could be* the trigger for a bout of CFS, we suspect that *anything* that reminds a thick boundary person of an earlier, unresolved trauma will put the bodymind gears into motion.

Here's a metaphor that should be helpful. Think of the city of New Orleans, laid low in August 2005 by Hurricane Katrina. It was a metropolis whose aging infrastructure was easily overwhelmed by the surging waters. This effectively is what happens during the upwelling that is CFS. The bodymind is in one sense liberated but in another sense overwhelmed. Memory ceases to function right, sleep is hard to come by, balance is impaired, numbness, headaches, odd tingling sensations come and go without warning. Even the smallest actions require effort, and such effort both exhausts and pains. It is quite like being, as Griffin described, in "a dilapidated house where every system fails" and the power is gone. In reality, *the power is being restored,* but the process will be lengthy and tax the individual's patience and determination as nothing else could.

PTSD: A NEW VIEW

Let's contrast the person afflicted with CFS with someone affected by PTSD. At first glance, they seem to be opposites: a mysterious malaise that portends who-knows-what (CFS) versus a highly immediate, riveting "replay" of a terrifying event that's all too clear (PTSD). Furthermore, whereas the person with CFS may have a tough time getting to sleep, the person with PTSD may be awoken by nightmares. And while the CFS sufferer is likely to ignore her or his needs while carrying out a project or serving others, the person with PTSD is prone to feeling irritable, to being overtaken by sudden bouts of anger, and to displaying hypervigilance and hyperarousal.[18]

The fascinating thing about PTSD (though obviously distressing to the person burdened by it) is how the individual essentially relives the traumatic event as though it's a clear and present danger. The sights, sounds, smells, and—especially—feelings are brought into visceral reality. What could cause this reexperiencing to be so vivid when, for someone suffering under the weight of CFS, it's unclear what, if anything, lurks behind the fog?

The concept of boundaries allows us to evaluate PTSD in an entirely new way. Let's start by viewing it as a thin boundary condition. A fair amount of biological evidence supports this proposition. First, activation of the HPA axis is higher in people suffering from PTSD than in people who live with CFS.[19] The level of serotonin—a neurotransmitter that influences HPA activity—is also low in PTSD sufferers compared with individuals experiencing CFS.[20] Additionally, cerebral blood flow in people undergoing a PTSD "flashback" is markedly higher compared with people who have CFS.[21]

The reactive nature of the thin boundary person with PTSD is captured by the following remark from a combat veteran. The smell of gunpowder, he said, not only makes him feel hot, "It's as if my whole metabolism changes."[22] The experience is intense as well as instantaneous.

We surmise the following is taking place in cases of PTSD. When a thin boundary person is physically assaulted, the stirred up feelings don't just recede into the bodymind, as they do with someone who has a thick boundary. They form a tight knot, a kind of stone in the energetic stream. (Contrast this by picturing CFS as a condition in which the feelings are walled off or dammed up.) When the person is reminded of the original event, the feeling "current" pushes the stone to the surface—where it evokes a frightening replay of the trauma in the here and now.

Ultimately, *boundaries make the difference.* CFS gathers force out of the awareness of a thick boundary person. But with PTSD, the person's thinner boundaries allow for a much more immediate retrieval of the dissociated energy—so much so that the replayed experience feels almost identical to the original trauma.

IRRITABLE BOWEL SYNDROME

Let's look now at another "syndrome," irritable bowel syndrome or IBS. People with IBS—10 percent to 15 percent of the U.S. population and nearly three-quarters of them women—experience chronic gastrointestinal pain and discomfort (also known by the medical term colitis).[23] Astonishingly, half of them have a history of being physically or sexually abused.[24] Others experienced such childhood traumas as a parental divorce, a major illness or accident, or the death of a loved one.[25] But IBS also runs in families, suggesting a genetic basis for the illness.[26]

IBS is demonstrably a thin boundary condition. First and foremost, sufferers are often described as "overly anxious" and even "driven"—a clear difference from the resolute, responsible personality of the CFS sufferer.[27] Second, IBS often co-occurs with seasonal allergies and allergic eczema; allergy itself is a marker of the thin boundary personality.[28] Furthermore, people with IBS are more likely to suffer from fibromyalgia and migraine (also thin boundary conditions, as we'll see).[29]

Another important difference between IBS and thick boundary conditions relates to serotonin (95 percent of which is actually found in the gut rather than in the "first brain").[30] The level of serotonin in IBS patients (and, for that matter, fibromyalgia sufferers) is low compared with individuals experiencing CFS.[31] While serotonin is far from the sole actor in activation or suppression of the HPA axis, the difference here points toward a meaningful distinction in boundary type among these conditions.

FIBROMYALGIA

People affected by fibromyalgia syndrome, or FMS, complain that specific parts of their body are painful to the touch. They may also have a generalized feeling of muscle tenderness and "aching all over." FMS is often categorized as a rheumatoid disorder because the features are similar. Indeed, the word fibromyalgia is an amalgam of *fibro* (for the soft tissues under the skin), *myo* (for the muscles), and *algia* (for pain). However, other types of complaints are often present: tingling sensations, localized numbness, headache, fatigue, difficulty sleeping, anxiety, and irritable bowel symptoms.[32]

So, while FMS may appear to be a musculoskeletal illness, it is better viewed as a more generalized disturbance of how the central nervous system processes pain.[33] This would explain why many people with FMS not only experience pain in response to touch and position but also (like migraine sufferers) to stimuli such as noise and light as well as changes in temperature and humidity. Their discomfort is anything but imaginary. People with FMS have been found to harbor elevated levels of substance P, a neurotransmitter involved in pain processing.[34]

The evidence suggests that FMS is a thin boundary condition, akin to IBS and migraine. We noted earlier that people with IBS often have symptoms of FMS; the converse is also true.[35] Likewise, people who suffer from migraine are more likely to have symptoms of FMS and vice versa.[36] FMS and IBS patients also have in common a lower level of serotonin, betokening greater activation of the HPA stress response system.[37] Additionally, two studies have tied FMS symptoms to PTSD, which we've posited is another thin boundary condition.[38]

While people with FMS may have some genetic predisposition, it seems clear that, in many cases, childhood trauma sensitizes them by lowering the HPA "bar."[39] As a rough analogy, think of what happens in cases of whiplash. People involved in even low-speed accidents will often clench their muscles and brace themselves for an anticipated impact. The effort expended in "hunkering down" can result in persistant neck or back pain.[40] In a parallel way, significant *emotional* stressors could cause a thin boundary person to clench his or her feeling energy, compressing it and setting the stage for later FMS symptoms.

A PERSONAL REMINISCENCE

One of the authors of this book experienced FMS when he was at the early crest of conventionally defined professional success. First came insomnia for many months, often with a feeling of being "on fire" when trying to fall asleep. At other times, a numbness or fogginess would settle in, making it virtually impossible for him to decide what to wear, what to eat, or where to go. Physician colleagues could find nothing wrong and attributed his problems to "burning the candle at both ends."

The candle almost burned itself out completely before he sought alternative medical treatments, having studied them for many years as an impartial observer. Chinese medicine practitioners had no trouble making a diagnosis: an imbalance of *qi,* or vital energy. With a series of acupuncture treatments, massage, and some extraordinary energy healing sessions (addressed in chapter 8), the pain and numbness receded. To this day, some amount of chronic pain remains in his lower legs—a constant reminder of what can happen when one permits others to define success and fulfillment in life.

A MIX OF CONDITIONS

Some people have a combination of thick and thin boundary conditions; for example, they experience CFS along with FMS. If you're such a person, what aspects of our discussion can you apply to your situation?

First off, it's likely that when you take the Boundary Questionnaire (BQ), your score will not fall on either extreme of the spectrum. Your thick boundary illness (more of which will be discussed in chapter 5) can be appropriately viewed as a sort of benchmark in your life at present. The fact that you have another illness (or illnesses) associated with the thin boundary profile suggests that you are more naturally a thin boundary person who, nevertheless, is dealing with an emotional challenge. Perhaps the onset of your CFS (or other thick boundary condition) coincided with this feeling-laden issue, or perhaps an accumulation of stressors was responsible. In any event, it's entirely possible that the chronic fatigue belies your more intrinsic thin boundary characteristics. If you can get at the source of whatever emotional "wrestling match" is taking place under the surface, you may find that, in due course, your personality traits become thinner and your BQ score shifts accordingly.

For someone whose thick boundary illness does *not* coincide with other, thin boundary conditions, it is likely that he or she is constitutionally thicker, and will score significantly thicker on the BQ.

SUMMING UP

Thomas Jefferson once remarked that, for the civic body, "the price of freedom is eternal vigilance." Our bodyminds often live out the truth of that concept. When we realize how psychosomatic illness can reflect the forces within us that remain on alert, it's clear that emotional freedom can, often enough, be gained only at a price.

We've seen that, for a variety of chronic conditions, intense, emotional experiences—particularly in childhood—reverberate "under the radar" throughout one's life. Whether we view the process through a strictly scientific lens (focusing on the HPA stress-handling system) or by examining the ways that the energy of feeling flows within us, it's clear that intensive experiences have various health effects *depending on personality type.*

In the following chapter, we'll look more closely at the connection between boundaries and how we feel our feelings—or don't, as the case may be.

Chapter 5

FEELINGS ON HOLD

Depression, Hypertension, Migraine, and Phantom Pain

Can your bodymind speak? As we've seen so far in this book, the answer is an unequivocal yes. Remember, in chapter 2, the woman who broke out in hives when reminded of her domineering mother-in-law; the lady whose facial rash seemed to reflect a long-standing concern over "facing" her husband's illness; and the psychologist who felt her clients' concerns manifested though her own aches and pains during therapy. In the last chapter, we gathered the truth of the adage "When we ignore what matters most to us, it will become the matter within us." Unresolved childhood traumas, we found, can become manifest in the adult conditions of chronic fatigue, irritable bowel, and fibromyalgia.

Clearly, some feelings are more likely to register in our awareness than others. Those that threaten to be overwhelming are often shunted aside, repressed, or denied. The uncoupling of ourselves from our feelings is termed *dissociation*. Everyone dissociates from time to time—it's quite natural and quite human. (If you've ever gotten lost in a good book or become engrossed in a task, odds are you've dissociated. You got so "into it" that you lost track of time, perhaps even of basic needs such as hunger or thirst.) Everyone dissociates, thin boundary or thick and every shade in between. But, in the case of strong feelings that are forced underground, the energy inherent in those feelings—their *e-motion*—will not be denied. Even as simple a mechanism as a blush represents an instance of a feeling "speaking out." A migraine, we also noted in chapter 2, can similarly reflect the dawning awareness of a particularly intense feeling or set of feelings.

In this chapter, we'll look more closely at conditions in which dissociation plays a key role. Just as CFS, PTSD, IBS, and FMS are characteristic of a boundary type, so are the conditions we'll assess here. We'll finish by looking at a widespread health concern in our modern society—depression—and find that, for a very important reason, it's independent of any particular boundary type. *Anyone can become depressed.* The whys and wherefores, though, can teach us a lot about how feelings work.

HYPERTENSION: A STORM BENEATH THE SURFACE

Psychologist James J. Lynch has spent decades investigating stress, hypertension, and heart disease. At his clinic in the late 1970s and early 1980s, he realized that some of his patients were demonstrating an amazing form of dissociation: their hands would be incredibly cold (20 degrees below normal); their hearts would be beating twice as fast as normal (125 beats per minute); their blood pressure would register exceedingly low (98/50) or stunningly high (210/125)—and all the while, they would appear pleasantly unaware that anything odd was happening to them.[1]

Lynch began to puzzle out the evidence. While these people claimed not to be feeling anything out of the ordinary (or much at all), their bodies were evidently "speaking" volumes. This peculiar form of expression seemed to manifest when they addressed major emotional issues in their lives, such as when a woman began to talk about how she hated her mother or a man described his father's death and his mother's stroke. In each of these cases, Lynch's patients would maintain a wan smile or a controlled monotone, betraying no ripple on a placid bodily surface . . . except that the monitors to which they were connected would show huge fluctuations in heart rate, blood pressure, and skin surface blood flow. In Lynch's words, it was as if they "were expending an amount of cardiovascular energy more appropriate for runners in a marathon than for people chatting quietly in an office."[2]

The fact that emotional issues seemed to rile these people up is the key. Recall the term *dispositional energy* from chapter 1, relating to one's ability to draw on a reservoir of vigor and active engagement with the world. We noted there's evidence that people with high dispositional energy are less likely to be affected by stress and inflammatory diseases such as rheumatoid arthritis, heart attacks, and strokes. Lynch's patients were in the opposite camp. Those illnesses were the very ones to which they were prone. Was their reservoir of energy any lower? It depends on how you look at it. They clearly had lots of energy, but it was "under wraps"—locked away, denied, consciously inaccessible. Hypertension was part and parcel of who they were, but they didn't realize it. *This is the thick boundary personality at work.*

Here's a case in point—a patient of Lynch he refers to as Patty.

At age 33, she seemed to have hardly a care in the world. Bright, effervescent, witty and pleasant, she would have been a perfect hostess for a daytime television show . . . Nor did she look as though she had endured a succession of emotional traumas in her life . . . it was difficult to interact with Patty and to appreciate fully the depths of her suffering.[3]

Her cardiovascular system, though, "could change in remarkable ways without the slightest awareness" on her part. In a typical treatment session with Lynch, she appeared to be in an upbeat mood as she spoke light-heartedly of some of the problems she had experienced the previous week, even as the monitors she was wearing showed her heart rate racing along at 110 to 130 beats per minute—faster than if she were jogging—and her blood pressure dipping to a low of 95/60. This paradoxical situation could only come about if her blood pressure had dropped precipitously and her heart was racing to compensate in an effort to keep her blood pressure up and prevent her from fainting outright.

As Lynch relates, Patty would discuss highly volatile subjects—her husband's having left her and remarrying, his failure to pay her alimony or provide emotional support for their son—in a calm, pleasant way, even as her hand temperature never rose above the room temperature of 72 degrees.[4] The coldness of her hands indicates the dramatic changes of Patty's blood circulation, with blood being shunted away from the skin as a result of her blood pressure dropping and her heart speeding up in response. The contrast between Patty's internal chaos and her outward demeanor could not have been more pronounced.

Indeed, at one point Lynch suggested that she resembled no one so much as the Mona Lisa, whose captivating half-smile distracts observers from noting her bluish white hands folded unobtrusively in her lap. "Who should I listen to, Patty?" he asked. "The woman with the lovely smile and happy-sounding voice, or the woman whose heart races . . . and whose hands are freezing cold?" Faced with this line of questioning, as well as the physiological gauges tracing their lines before her, Patty then "stopped smiling and fell silent. . . . Finally she remarked with a pained, semi-forced smile, 'I guess I let the insides do the crying for me.'"[5]

Not only hypertension, but panic attacks also may be indicative of thick boundary functioning in which threatening feelings have gone "underground" within the bodymind. A recent study monitored people who were prone to panic attacks, finding that these patients experienced symptoms well before they became consciously aware of being panicked. For example, a person's carbon dioxide level would register as abnormally low (indicative of chronic hyperventilation) up to 47 minutes before he or she literally pressed a panic button on the waist pack monitoring their physiology. For these people, the attack seemed to come out of the blue, though their bodies showed unmistakable evidence of strong feelings.[6]

Individuals who have hypertension or chronic cardiovascular problems tend toward a remarkable lack of awareness concerning their dramatic shifts in blood pressure, heart rate, and skin conductance when emotional subjects are brought up.[7] On a plainly physical level, those issues are obviously causing the person turmoil. Yet the individual will tend to sense only an emptiness, detachment, or obliviousness. The discrepancy between the thick boundary person's physical symptoms and surface calm is a measure of how dissociated she or he is from the intensive feelings lurking within. Their bodymind, however, will not be truly silenced.

RHEUMATOID ARTHRITIS

Rheumatoid arthritis is a disease characterized by painful swelling of the tissue lining the joints, typically the small joints of the hands and feet. Unlike the wear and tear of osteoarthritis, rheumatoid arthritis is an autoimmune disorder where the immune system mistakenly attacks the person's own tissue. Its symptoms can also include fever and fatigue.

Sometimes a person with rheumatoid arthritis resembles Patty, the thick boundary person we met above—someone skilled at hiding feelings from herself while her blood pressure, heart rate, or cold hands give her away.[8] Interestingly, rheumatoid arthritis is associated with issues of feeling "stuck," at least in the estimation of several perceptive clinicians. A person suffering from stiff or painfully swollen joints could well be describing her- or himself through comments such as "I'm in a bind," "I'm in a rut," "I can't get moving," or "I don't know what I want."[9] The illness effectively functions as a somatic metaphor—a physical representation of the sufferer's internal (if unacknowledged) experience.[10] Rather than embrace her or his own feelings and needs and do something about them, the person with rheumatoid arthritis tends to focus on other people and act upon *their* feelings and needs.

MIGRAINE, UP CLOSE AND PERSONAL

A fair way to differentiate the effects on different sides of the boundary spectrum—at least when strong feelings are dissociated—is the following. *While a thick boundary person has difficulty realizing that he or she is feeling anything significant, the thin boundary person has some awareness of the presence of the feelings but is slow to appreciate their intensity.*

Migraine headaches are a good illustration of this thin boundary dilemma. The fact that a migraine can be brought on by just about anything—an aroma, a noise, a food, glare, changing weather conditions—indicates that a thin boundary person is most likely to be affected. A migraine can also (as noted in chapter 2) be brought on by emotional upset. We had a memorable look into the dynamics of a therapist whose headaches occurred immediately after an emotionally devastating exchange in his office between a husband and a wife. Recall that the therapist "identified with everything" and was soon "blindsided" by the powerful combination of feelings.

Interestingly, the same counselor no longer suffers from migraines. He says he's come to "recognize the early signs . . . [and] transform these into feelings."[11] Once a person prone to migraine is able to acknowledge the buildup (and, if appropriate, respond to or express the feelings), the headache will, like a wave, crash over and recede.

Here's another illustration of how strong feelings can lead to a migraine. James Lance, a headache expert in Australia, relates the following story:

A patient of mine was having a heated argument with a girlfriend about the rebellious attitude he had towards his father when he had been a teenager, a subject that had distressed him in later years. At the height of the argument his vision started to blur, and soon he could see only the centre of objects. This tunnel vision lasted for about 10 minutes, after which his characteristic migraine headache developed. Some weeks later he was attending a cinema and found that the film dealt with the same problem of the father-son relationship that had always troubled him. Within a few minutes his vision misted over, and tunnel vision was again followed by a headache.[12]

Now, we are all affected by emotion in our lives, but not everyone suffers from migraine. Such headaches affect approximately thirty million Americans, 75 percent of whom are women. Migraines typically occur after puberty begins and diminish after the onset of menopause.[13] Presumably, then, the female sex hormones play a role. But new evidence suggests that nurture, as well as nature, could be decisive. A study published by the American Headache Society finds that childhood maltreatment, especially emotional abuse and neglect, are prevalent among migraine patients. The study asked over 17,000 migraineurs to report "adverse childhood experiences," such as being physically assaulted, witnessing domestic violence, and so on. The more such experiences that a person reported, the greater his or her likelihood of having frequent headaches.[14] It's a short step to infer that the hypothalamic-pituitary-adrenal (HPA) set point in these people has become lowered so that emotional strife results in severe headaches as they get older.

In sum, the picture we are developing is that of highly sensitive, thin boundary people who nonetheless are taken by surprise when strong feelings well up in the form of a migraine.

BLOOD FLOW IN MIGRAINE AND CFS

Biologically, migraine is a two-step process. In the lead-up phase, before the headache is experienced but when sufferers tend to feel depressed, irritable, or restless, serotonin levels are unusually high, constricting blood flow. Then, when the headache actually hits, serotonin levels drop sharply and the blood vessels dilate.[15]

Lynch relates these two phases to the patient's handling of emotion. If the person is going through a stressful period, blood flow to the extremities will be constricted; this condition can last for hours or days, according to Lynch. Finally, they relax a bit, and blood returns to the extremities, "all the more strongly for having been constricted." The blood vessels dilate and the migraine occurs.[16]

Blood flow is an emerging area of interest medically. Particularly for CFS, it is beginning to be studied avidly. Researchers have measured a distinct difference between the cerebral blood flow of their CFS patients and that of controls.[17] Even circulating blood volume appears to be lower among many CFS patients.[18] Whereas the normal adult body has approximately five quarts of blood, these people have 20 percent— or fully one quart—less.[19] David Bell, former chair of the CFS Advisory Committee of the U.S. Department of Health and Human Services, comments that he's "not found anyone with CFS who can keep their [blood] volume up. . . . For some reason the body does not want to accept a normal volume."[20] (Interestingly, in Chinese medicine, chronic fatigue is described as a deficiency of blood, as well as a deficiency of *qi*. The concept of qi and its relationship to chronic illness will be taken up in chapter 8.)

These findings indicate not hypertension but *hypo*tension among CFS patients. If our supposition about the flow of feeling in the bodymind is correct—and reduced blood flow in the brain and body is akin to reduced feeling flow—then people afflicted by CFS appear to be significantly thick boundary. That is, at least until their flow of feeling is restored and a healthier balance is attained.

DISSOCIATION IN ASTHMA AND ALLERGIES

We stated earlier that dissociation can play a role in anyone's chronic illness, whether the person is on the thick or thin side of the boundary spectrum. The effects are different because a thick boundary person tends not to be conversant with feelings in the first place, whereas a thin boundary person who is emotionally receptive may nonetheless "wall off" problematic feelings or recollections.

Asthma and allergies are a commonplace example of the latter process. Asthma, it has been suggested, may reflect or mask unresolved grief.[21] Whether or not this correspondence is correct in most or all cases, the condition itself is most likely thin boundary, as it is known to co-occur with migraine[22] and has even been linked to PTSD[23]—both of which are thin boundary conditions.

Many people, unfortunately, suffer from asthma and allergies together. Our first book, *The Spiritual Anatomy of Emotion*, offered intriguing evidence that allergies are similarly indicative of thin boundaries.[24] This makes intuitive sense because more in the external environment "gets" to a thin boundary person, and her or his bodymind will then overreact to it. Given the centrality of feelings to our sense of self, it is reasonable to suppose that an individual's dissociation from especially intense feelings will aggravate his or her tendency toward allergies.

PHANTOM PAIN: CONTRASTING CASES

A side-by-side view of how thick and thin boundaries work can be gained through the phenomenon of phantom pain. This is a challenging condition wherein people who have lost a limb will complain vigorously about strange sensations where their arm or leg, hand or foot used to be. "Cramping," "itching," "burning," and "shooting" pains are the adjectives most commonly used. In every case, the person is convinced that the limb (or whatever the body part may be) is still there. Sometimes the phantom sensations occur immediately after a patient's surgery; sometimes they manifest after weeks, months, or even years. In some cases they abate, only to return later. The phenomenon is quite common, affecting upwards of 70 percent of amputees.[25]

These cases have yet to be understood. But perhaps phantom pain can be explained through feelings and the energy they harbor. The first question we must pose is: What distinguishes the 30 percent of amputees who don't experience phantom pain from the majority who do? Similarly, why should some people's sensations come and go while others' remain constant? The answer might have to do with the extent to which feelings are dissociated in that person. *Someone who is chronically dissociated is much more likely to feel phantom pain,* in our estimation.

Initial evidence to this effect has been gathered by Eric Leskowitz, a Boston-based psychiatrist and energy healer who directs the Integrative Medicine Project at Spaulding Rehabilitation Hospital. Leskowitz has raised a number of intriguing issues on the possible relationship between stress, emotion, and the resolution of phantom limb pain. For example, he treated two patients whose reaction to their respective predicaments differed quite a bit. The first patient, "Mr. A," was

> a 37-year-old cargo loader, who lost his left leg just below the knee after suffering a massive crush injury when a cargo dolly jackknifed into his leg. He developed stump and phantom pain which was not responsive to two years of rehabilitation treatments, including . . . anti-depressants to treat his concurrent major depression. Formerly an avid athlete, he appeared to withdraw from life due to the loss of his old self-image as a hockey player and "tough guy." He was also quite invested in a Worker's Compensation suit against his former employer, which consumed much of his emotional energy.
>
> He described this process of releasing his pain as frightening to him. Somehow, he was holding onto the pain and preventing it from totally leaving his body. He realized that if he could no longer feel any pain in his phantom leg, he would have to experience the true absence of his leg for the first time since his injury . . . doing so would also involve accepting the fact that he would never play hockey again. He stated quite clearly that he was not ready to proceed with further energy healing, because he wasn't yet ready to accept his disability.[26]

Contrast this patient's reaction and outlook with that of another patient, "Ms. B,"

> a 65-year-old widow whose severe diabetic peripheral vascular disease necessitated a below-the-knee amputation of her right leg. However, she apparently misunderstood her surgeon's plans,

because she went into surgery with the expectation that only two of her toes would be removed (the painful and gangrenous ones). Needless to say, she was shocked to wake up and find her lower leg missing. Within hours of her [surgery], she developed phantom pain of the two toes she had expected to lose. . . . She proved to be a feisty yet trusting woman who was primarily upset that her esteemed surgeon had so misled her. Part of her psychotherapeutic work with me involved venting her frustration, and also communicating her distress directly to her surgeon. These conversations allowed her to feel as though a load was lifted from her shoulders. . . . [Later] the phantom pain dissipated . . . she was pain free for the first time since surgery.[27]

The differences between these two instances are striking. Mr. A desperately wished to retain his old self-image as the rough-and-ready hockey player, whereas Ms. B was able, after venting her anger and frustration, to accept her predicament.

To the extent, then, that a person can come to terms with his or her deepest feelings, dissociation—and phantom pain—will be reduced. We suggest that the 30 percent of amputees who *don't* suffer from phantom pain are thin boundary types who are more fluent in the language of feeling than thicker boundary people whose bodies, nevertheless, manage to speak for them.

ULCER: ANOTHER SHADE OF THICK BOUNDARY PAIN

A more prosaic thick boundary condition is that of ulcer. While an ulcer is typically something we associate with the stomach, our skin, especially skin directly overlying bone, can also become ulcerated. (An example is the bed sore.) Where stomach ulcers are concerned, we noted in chapter 3 that stress or anxiety presumably plays a role, because the *H. pylori* bacterium in the stomach lining associated with ulcer doesn't affect everyone equally. The overwhelming majority of people with *H. pylori* in their system don't develop a stomach ulcer, and other patients who *do* develop an ulcer don't even harbor the bacterium.[28]

Our contention is that thick boundary people are more likely to develop this condition. One intriguing clue is the association of ulcers with phantom pain. Some people who have had a hand, a foot, or a limb removed can feel an area of irritation—be it a skin ulcer, a bunion, or even a tight ring that had been around their finger—long after the surgery.[29] If, as we've proposed, phantom pain is more likely to be experienced by thick boundary people, an ulcer would be in the same category.

NOT KNOWING YOUR FEELINGS: ALEXITHYMIA

Language itself—even something said offhand—often provides an indication of someone's true thoughts or feelings. (Freudian slips are famous in this regard.) An interesting observation made by Lynch is how some of his patients would speak passively about their health conditions. An example: "The blood pressure really went up last week" (as opposed to "my" blood pressure went up). Lynch draws a contrast with how most of us would describe our blushing: "I blushed just now" versus "My face blushed" or "It blushed just now." The more impersonal language, he notes, marks a disconnect between our selves and our bodily states. A blush—or hypertension, or a migraine, or CFS—is not something you "have" but is an active part of *you*.[30] These conditions reflect your body-mind, and your bodymind is literally your self.

Independently, both Lynch and Ernest Hartmann (originator of the boundaries framework) use the term *alexithymia* to describe what might be going on. Alexithymia (pronounced "alex-uh-THIGH-me-yah") is a concept introduced by the late Harvard University psychiatrist Peter Sifneos in 1973 to describe people who seem not to understand that they have feelings or lack the words to identify those feelings.[31] The word derives from Greek: *a* for lack (as in apathy); *lexis* for word; and *thymos* for emotion. Sifneos applied the concept to people who either are troubled psychosomatically but who, like Patty, put on a happy face and claim they're all right or recount their most difficult life experiences impassively, as if what happened to them made little or no difference.[32]

Alexithymia offers a framework for understanding the emotional makeup of certain people. On the surface, it may appear similar to depression or autism spectrum disorder, two other conditions in which people have difficulty recognizing or articulating their feelings. In those cases, though, an observer probably wouldn't suggest that the autistic or depressed person doesn't *know* what he or she is feeling. People who are alexithymic, in contrast, have an interior life that seems impoverished. Their facial expressions are often wooden and their postures stiff (mirroring their internal state). They may recount what happened to them—a conversation, for example, or a meeting they had—in monotonous detail. But they'll never indicate that what happened to them *felt like* anything. Instead, the person who's alexithymic will "decode" what he or she might have been feeling from the comments of others and clues from his or her own body. For example, "I was clenching my fist and others around me seemed distressed, so perhaps I was angry."[33]

As you might expect, alexithymia is a strongly thick boundary condition. In Hartmann's words, people with alexithymia "[keep] things very separate and [do] not make many connections among their thoughts, feelings, images, etc."[34] Without a base of readily available feelings to draw upon, alexithymics have a bland imagination and little fantasy life to speak of. They are tied to concrete thinking and are typically unable to see the value of poetry or the point of figures of speech such as "a rolling stone gathers no moss."[35] Furthermore, alexithymics don't score well on dream recall, and the dreams they do remember are concerned with literal, practical issues. Their dreaming lacks the vividness and symbolic imagery of people who are toward the thin side of the boundary spectrum.[36]

In fact, people who are told they're alexithymic are unable to realize it.[37] For this reason, they don't respond well to traditional psychotherapy, which aims to bring subconscious feelings to light. Someone who is alexithymic has no apparent neuroses, no hidden conflicts to speak of. Fundamentally, the person seems "affect-less."[38]

It would be easy to conclude that people with alexithymia *have* no feelings—but that's not where the evidence leads. For one thing, their tendency to intellectualize and "keep things in place" (by tightening up their bodies or being highly organized) suggests an avid effort to keep threatening thoughts or feelings at bay.[39] Yet psychosomatic ailments do plague the alexithymic. Rashes, irritable bowel–type symptoms, chronic pain, chronic fatigue, asthma, migraine, and hypertension have all been documented.[40] Researchers have even noted an overlap between alexithymia and Asperger's disorder (a high-functioning form of autism).[41]

Considering its thick boundary nature, we suspect that alexithymia will be shown to be closely related to a condition such as chronic fatigue syndrome—and there is some evidence to support this proposition. One study found that a group of CFS patients had difficulty expressing themselves because of reduced blood flow to the parts of the brain controlling vocabulary.[42] However, as noted above, certain people with alexithymia end up contracting thin boundary ailments. It may be that these individuals are "thinner" by nature but have been raised in a resolutely thick boundary environment, thus complicating the picture. A significant emotional challenge in the here and now—an accident, for example, or the breakout of a relationship—might prompt bodymind symptoms that are a mixture of thin and thick. In any event, one thing is clear: boundaries provide an entirely new way to evaluate this condition.

How Does Alexithymia Begin?

Similar to the other bodymind conditions we've explored in this book, alexithymia presumably owes to a combination of nature and nurture. For example, when a questionnaire assessing alexithymia was given to nearly eight thousand pairs of twins in Denmark, the results suggested that genetics would account for about one-third of the cases and environmental influences would account for the rest.[43] It's also been found that people who have suffered a traumatic head injury are much more likely to exhibit the condition.[44]

On the nurture side of things, there's another, more mundane cause to consider. Lynch suggests that emotionally unaware parents effectively teach the same ignorance of feelings to their children. "If mothers or fathers cannot sense their own feelings," he writes, "how can they teach their offspring about feelings or sense the feelings of these children? . . . Like their parents, the children will react inside their bodies without exhibiting any external signs of stress." So a mother who is used to cold hands when feeling upset, will, by her own example, set the stage for reduced blood flow—and cold extremities—in her daughter as *she* dissociates from threatening feelings.[45] Not being able to detect feeling in oneself or others becomes a fateful family circle.

Another school of thought suggests that people who are alexithymic become that way because they cannot bear to have their emotional forays frustrated by caregivers. If a child's expression of emotions finds no validation on the part of others, so the explanation goes, he or she will be threatened by unbearable tension—and to become alexithymic is to foreclose on the possibility of such tensions arising. Never owning up to one's feelings— even to the fact that one *has* feelings—is a way for the developing child to protect him- or herself and to leave any emotional interactions alone. Inexpressiveness will then become that person's way of being in the world.[46]

A Way with(out) Words

And what of the *lex* part of alexithymia—the lack of words for feelings? Earlier in this book, we suggested that emotion was a bit like a foreign language for thick boundary people. Keeping with this analogy, we might say that *the alexithymic is almost illiterate.* How such a lack probably takes root is, again, nicely captured by Lynch:

> When first taught, human communication involves a parent's reassurance that the child's emotional experience is real . . . the parent begins to teach the child words to distinguish various bodily feelings—*hurt, lonely, loving, sad, happy.* Each word given to the child, and anchored in a particular bodily feeling, thus forms the foundation upon which a child builds the capacity to communicate his or her feelings to others.[47]

This "language of the heart" gives us a working vocabulary to represent what we're feeling inside—and a means to intuit what others are feeling. Alas, people with alexithymia are severely limited in this regard. While anyone, regardless of boundary type, can dissociate from his or her feelings, the crucial distinction with alexithymia is that others harbor the means to *regain use of that vocabulary.* When a person blushes, has a migraine, or experiences IBS, CFS, FMS, phantom pain, PTSD, or any of the other health conditions we have been considering, he or she at least knows something is amiss. The alexithymic typically does not—unless the individual manages, eventually, to overcome the feeling deficit and "come home" to his or her emotional core.

DEPRESSION KNOWS NO BOUNDARIES

The final health condition we'll address in this chapter is depression. It is widespread, the latest figures showing that more than one in seven adults in the United States has experienced a major depressive episode.[48] Furthermore, depression frequently accompanies many of the chronic illnesses we have discussed.

It's exceedingly difficult for medical science to tease out where those other conditions end and depression begins. Many researchers once believed that psychosomatic ailments were brought on by the person's depression. However, more recent studies suggest that people can become depressed as a *consequence* of the illnesses with which they're afflicted.[49] Especially for a person whose health complaints are written off as "all in their head," whose symptoms cannot be easily pegged to a known illnesses, and whose reports of suffering are met by friends, family, and caregivers with disbelief, it's easy to see how depression could follow.

Where, then, does depression fit on the boundary scale? We find that depression may actually be independent of thick-thin boundary classification. It can affect anyone based on one's response to a significant loss or disappointment; specifically, how such a loss (real or perceived) affects the person's self-worth, and the extent to which she or he is able to rebound.[50]

Some people, by virtue of their genetic inheritance as well as upbringing, demonstrate a reaction that's in proportion to the turn of events—they're genuinely sad but gradually feel better and are able to move on. Others react with intensive and lasting sadness that plays out, in various forms and guises, years after the original experience. Their self-worth, it seems, has taken such a serious blow that they never truly recover. Indeed, one can achieve great things and be celebrated in others' eyes and still regard oneself as unworthy of happiness or success. The weight of such depression can be extremely difficult to dislodge.

From the standpoint of feelings, it's been said that depression is a matter of anger or disappointment turned inward—relating to a time when the person had no choice but to accept what fate had in store. We suspect this explanation is correct in virtually all cases. If the person with depression had a healthy coping style, he or she would rage against the source of the loss (like King Lear on the stormy heath) or find a suitable outlet for his or her indignation. Instead, the depressive's self-image takes a hit. Legitimate anger and resentment are accompanied or replaced by a sense of being unworthy, even of shame or self-loathing.

This process bears some similarity to alexithymia because, when the switch occurs, the individual may be unaware of it. Anger is thoroughly and instantaneously displaced, supplanted for the foreseeable future by low self-regard and a generalized numbness to the transformation. The person's dispositional energy will be low because the feelings are walled off and, with them, the reservoir of bodymind energy.

If this description sounds a bit like our conception of chronic fatigue syndrome, a distinction is in order. Depression is primarily a *pattern to be overcome* rather than a set of *memories to be integrated*. Here is the difference. Whereas, in CFS, long dormant energy becomes forcefully reintegrated into the self, in depression the conscious self is actively seeking to keep feelings at bay that it regards as threatening—

and *consciousness holds the upper hand*. This is Freud's classic repression. It's a more active "hold" on feelings than in CFS, hypertension, migraine, irritable bowel syndrome, phantom pain, fibromyalgia, or any of the other conditions we've been considering. In all of these other cases, the dissociated feelings make themselves quite vigorously known. The depressed person, however, is in an ongoing funk. He or she can be despairingly sad most of the time, happy at other times, but the dominant feeling is "blah." It is more of an existential pain than a piercing, physical discomfort. That's because the underlying feelings are on "mute." Depression, therefore, requires a more active, conscious effort to overcome, while the other conditions principally call for the person to be open to a reconciliation with the displaced or relegated feelings.

TREATING DEPRESSION

In chapter 7, we'll suggest various complementary and alternative therapies that are effective at relieving depression and restoring a healthier flow of feeling. One thing we do *not* recommend is an exclusive reliance on drugs such as Prozac and Zoloft. These medications, which increase the level of serotonin in the brain, may be helpful to some people, but they do nothing to address issues of *feeling* in the body. In fact, one consequence of their use is that feeling may actually be numbed—a development not always welcomed by the sufferer. Or these drugs may give the person a lift (which, of course, is their aim). If the underlying emotional issues are left unaddressed, however, that energy uplift may only serve to amplify the individual's lack of self-esteem or general sense of hopelessness. This paradox is especially a concern if the person is suicidal.

Even in depression, the bodymind has ways to protect the self: if you can't mobilize the energy to do anything at all, you can't do anything harmful to yourself. (There are too many cases where someone who is depressed—whether an adolescent or an adult—is thoughtlessly prescribed Prozac, without being given supportive therapy, and suddenly commits suicide.[51]) Such drugs boost a person's serotonin level without dealing with the emotional dynamic underlying the depression. This pill is obviously far from the ideal way to handle a potentially life-threatening illness.

The issues that inevitably loom large in depression—a person's early relationship with caregivers, an unexpected or traumatic experience, the conception the individual has about the value of his or her own life—have at least as much to do with the heart as the head. Rather than "listening to Prozac" (as suggested by a blithe, popular book of the same name) and medicating only the symptoms of the illness, we ought to *listen to the depression* and the message conveyed by its symptoms. The "blah" and the despair of depression are signs that something is seriously amiss inside. If we fail to attend to them, if we fail to explore their deeper meaning, the person inside will never truly be discovered.[52]

Chapter 6

FINDING YOUR BOUNDARY TYPE

You probably have a good idea whether you're on the thin or thick side of the boundary spectrum by now, if not from the first couple of chapters of this book, which presented the boundary concept, then from the last two chapters, which delved into particular chronic conditions. Before you take the short Boundary Questionnaire (BQ), however, allow us a brief recap.

THE BOUNDARY QUESTIONNAIRE

The BQ was developed by Ernest Hartmann, M.D., a dream researcher at Tufts University, based on research he conducted in the 1980s. Since then, more than five thousand people have taken the BQ and more than one hundred research papers have been published on it.[1]

The full version, which includes 145 questions, can be found in appendix A. The short form is presented here since it captures the essential information to enable you to assess your boundary type. The full BQ allows you a more in-depth appreciation of where you fall on the boundary spectrum according to items grouped into a dozen different categories, reflecting themes such as Interpersonal, Thoughts/Feelings/Moods, Childhood/Adolescence/Adult, and Sleep/Dream/Waking. So, one can be a thin or thick boundary person overall and score different places along the boundary spectrum within these categories. No one is reducible to a single spot on the boundary spectrum. Each of us is likely to be thin in some respects, thick in others.[2]

Moreover, where we are on the spectrum is not, in any sense, fixed for life. People tend to acquire thicker boundaries as they age but, obviously, everyone is different. Some people may develop thinner boundaries as they get older as a result of their unique experiences. A person's boundaries can even become thicker or thinner based on the medications he or she takes or depending on how tired the person happens to be.[3] Still, as a general personality trait, your boundary type won't vary too much from day to day or year to year.

The short form of the BQ is presented here. It's all of eighteen questions and usually takes less than ten minutes to complete and score. For anyone wishing a quick way to assess her or his boundary type, the short form BQ is the most direct route.

Please note: while the statements are phrased in a general way, none of them is meant as a value judgment. There are no right or wrong responses. Consider these statements merely as prompts intended to sound you out on where you are right now in your life.

That being said, please rate each of the statements from 0 to 4. A rating of 0 indicates "not at all" or "not at all true of me," whereas a rating of 4 indicates "yes, definitely" or "very true of me." Try to respond to all of the statements as quickly as you can.

SHORT FORM BOUNDARY QUESTIONNAIRE

1. My feelings blend into one another.   0 1 2 3 4

2. I am very close to my childhood feelings.   0 1 2 3 4

3. I am easily hurt.   0 1 2 3 4

4. I spend a lot of time daydreaming, fantasizing, or in reverie.   0 1 2 3 4

5. I like stories that have a definite beginning, middle, and end.   0 1 2 3 4

6. A good organization is one in which all the lines of responsibility are precise and clearly established.   0 1 2 3 4

7. There should be a place for everything, with everything in its place.   0 1 2 3 4

8. Sometimes it's scary when one gets too involved with another person.   0 1 2 3 4

9. A good parent has to be a bit of a child too.   0 1 2 3 4

10. I can easily imagine myself as an animal or what it might be like to be an animal.   0 1 2 3 4

11. When something happens to a friend of mine or to a lover, it is almost as if it happened to me.   0 1 2 3 4

12. When I work on a project, I don't like to tie myself down to a definite outline. I rather like to let my mind wander.   0 1 2 3 4

13. In my dreams, people sometimes merge into each other or become other people.   0 1 2 3 4

14. I believe I am influenced by forces that no one can understand.   0 1 2 3 4

15. There are no sharp dividing lines between normal people, people with problems, and people who are considered psychotic or crazy.   0 1 2 3 4

16. I am a down-to-earth, no-nonsense kind of person.   0 1 2 3 4

17. I think I would enjoy being some kind of creative artist.   0 1 2 3 4

18. I have had the experience of someone calling me or speaking my name and not being sure whether it was really happening or whether I was imagining it.   0 1 2 3 4

OBTAINING YOUR SCORE

To obtain your score, simply add up the scores (0–4) for all the statements—
except that the scores for questions 5, 6, 7, and 16 are scored backward
(i.e., for these questions an answer of "0" is scored as 4, "1" is scored as 3, "2"
is scored as 2, "3" is scored as 1, and "4" is scored as 0).

Scores below 30 are considered definitely "thick" and scores above 42 are considered definitely "thin." See where you are on the spectrum below:

THICK BOUNDARY----------------------**MIDDLE**------------------------**THIN BOUNDARY**

0	9	18	27	36	45	54	63	72

INTERESTING CORRELATIONS

Boundary type turns out to have a relationship with several topics we'll examine briefly here: the Myers-Briggs Type Indicator (MBTI); one's chosen occupation and other demographics; one's perception of her or his own boundary type; and the efficacy of placebos.

Myers-Briggs Type Indicator

The MBTI is a well-known personality assessment tool (it may be the world's most widely used). A person is scored via four pairs of opposites: Extraversion-Introversion, Sensing-Intuition, Thinking-Feeling, and Judgment-Perception. A four-letter code indicates the person's preference within each of the pairs. Someone whose type is ESTJ, for example, leans toward Extraversion (E), Sensing (S), Thinking (T), and Judgment (J), whereas someone whose type is INFP is inclined toward Introversion (I), Intuition (N), Feeling (F), and Perception (P).

A definite relationship has been shown between thin boundaries and Intuition and between thick boundaries and Sensing. To a lesser degree, thin boundaries are associated with Feeling and thick boundaries with Thinking. Also to a lesser extent, thin boundaries are associated with Perception and thick boundaries with Judgment. No correlation has been found between either boundary type and Introversion or Extraversion.[4] So an intuitive, sensitive, thin boundary person is just as apt to be outgoing as a questioning, fact-based, thick boundary person is to be reticent.

Demographics

Overall, people who take the BQ score all across the spectrum, similar to a bell-type curve. Women, however, tend to score significantly thinner than men, and older people generally score slightly thicker than younger people.[5]

Interestingly—though you may or may not fit the profile—people in certain professions have scored markedly thinner or thicker than people in other jobs. In the thin category are artists, musicians, and fashion models. In the thick category are naval officers, salespeople, and lawyers.[6]

Perception of Own and Other Boundary Type

As one might expect, people tend to consider their own boundary type desirable and may disparage qualities associated with the "other" type. Thin boundary people, for example, see themselves as exciting, creative, and innovative but can look upon those with thick boundaries as dull, rigid, and unimaginative. Thick boundary people, on the other hand, view themselves as solid, reliable, and persevering while sometimes considering those with thin boundaries as flaky, far out, and unreliable.[7] What can we say but *vive la différence!*

Placebo Effect

One important way of characterizing a distinctly thin boundary person is that he or she is open to experience.[8] It makes sense, therefore, that studies have found a correlation between thin boundaries and three personality traits: suggestibility, hypnotizability, and absorption (a measure of the extent to which someone can become enmeshed in an experience).[9]

Since the ability of placebos to effect a cure is mediated by these same traits, one could reasonably suppose that thinner boundary people would gain more benefit from placebos than thicker boundary people. This subject deserves further study because scientists do not know definitively why some people benefit more from placebos than others.[10] The issue, though, takes us directly into the next chapter and the question "Which therapeutic approaches work best for my boundary type?"

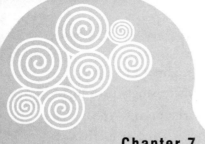

Chapter 7

FINDING YOUR REMEDY

Chronic health conditions affect a vast number of people—and the numbers in every case are rising. Just take a look:

- One out of four Americans suffers from asthma or allergies.[1] About one-third of that group is primarily affected by asthma.[2] Allergy itself is the fifth leading chronic disease in the United States.[3]
- Approximately 30% of adults in the United States suffer from hypertension, also known as high blood pressure. The numbers are higher for Europe.[4]
- About 12% of Americans suffer from migraine.[5] The percentage for women (17%) is higher.[6]
- Fibromyalgia afflicts 10 million Americans.[7] . . . chronic fatigue syndrome disrupts the lives of more than 1 million people in the United States[8] . . . and anywhere from 6% to 15% of the adult population in Canada, the United States, and the United Kingdom is estimated to have irritable bowel syndrome.[9]
- About 10% of women and 5% of men have had post-traumatic stress disorder at one time or another.[10]
- One in seven adults in the United States experiences a major depression during his or her lifetime.[11]

Taken together, these figures are staggering. Conventional medicine is overwhelmed, often ineffective, and patients are increasingly turning to complementary and alternative medicine (CAM) for treatment. The most recent estimate (for 2007) is that 38 percent of American adults spent nearly $34 billion out-of-pocket on approaches such as hypnosis, acupuncture, biofeedback, guided imagery, meditation, and yoga.[12] People are plainly searching for new ways to relieve their difficulties, especially as they see "one size fits all" medicine as uncaring and unresponsive to their particular needs. Conventional medicine is also rising exorbitantly in cost, complications, and complexity, so CAM approaches often provide a simple, cost-effective, and low-risk alternative.

This chapter considers seven of the best-documented CAM treatments for these conditions. But, consistent with our theme that people differ according to boundary type, some people will derive greater benefit from certain treatments than will other people. Put another way, *just as thin boundary and thick boundary people differ in the types of chronic illnesses to which they are susceptible, the types of CAM approaches that work best for them also differ.* A major goal of this book is to put this information into your hands, so that you can make an informed choice of which CAM treatments are right for you.

TREATMENTS FOR YOUR BOUNDARY TYPE

The "Super Seven" treatments we'll consider are

- hypnosis
- acupuncture
- biofeedback
- meditation and yoga (considered together)
- guided imagery
- relaxation and stress reduction

The Super Seven are not the only CAM therapies in use, of course.

We delve into these in particular because each is a well-established, safe, and effective treatment that is widely available and that's demonstrated proven, positive results for the medical conditions considered in this book.

Knowing what we do about boundaries—especially that people on the thin side of the boundary spectrum are better able to identify their feelings than are people on the thick side—we can project that thin boundary types will typically respond better to an *imagery-based* approach such as hypnosis or guided imagery. Thick boundary types, on the other hand, should respond well to more *hands-on* approaches such as acupuncture and biofeedback. And everyone can benefit to varying degrees from a practice that facilitates *relaxation,* be it meditation, yoga, or mindfulness-based stress reduction.

Through a survey of all available evidence, these expectations are generally on target. A few of our findings merit further exploration, however:

- Relaxation-based approaches, it turns out, work better for a number of the thick boundary conditions—because the dissociated feelings underlying them may require relaxation first, in order for the person to be receptive to the possibility that feelings are even at play.
- Biofeedback works at least as well for thin boundary conditions as for thick. Thin boundary people appreciate the instantaneous readouts that biofeedback provides, substantiating the associated feelings they need to address.
- Acupuncture works well for conditions across the boundary spectrum. (The reasons will be explored in the next chapter.)

The charts below indicate the effectiveness of the Super Seven for each of the Dozen Discomforts addressed in this book. We use a 1–5 scale, with 1 being "minimally effective," 3 being "moderately effective," and 5 being "highly effective." Where no number appears, it means that data were insufficient to support an evaluation.

The results presented here are drawn from coauthor Dr. Marc Micozzi's twenty years of experience reviewing and compiling thousands of studies for his textbook, *Fundamentals of Complementary and Alternative Medicine,* now in its fourth edition.[13] This textbook is considered the standard reference for physicians and scientists practicing and researching CAM treatments. However, an *analysis of CAM therapies according to boundary type has never before been undertaken; you, the reader, are the beneficiary.*

THICK BOUNDARY CONDITIONS

DISORDER	HYPNOSIS	ACUPUNCTURE	BIOFEEDBACK	MEDITATION/ YOGA	GUIDED IMAGERY	STRESS REDUCTION
Rheumatoid Arthritis		3	3	4		3
CFS		3	3	3	3	
Hypertension	2	1	4	5	2	4
Phantom Pain	1	4	2	2		
Psoriasis	2		3			
Ulcer						3

THIN BOUNDARY CONDITIONS

DISORDER	HYPNOSIS	ACUPUNCTURE	BIOFEEDBACK	MEDITATION/ YOGA	GUIDED IMAGERY	STRESS REDUCTION
Asthma/ Allergies	4	5	4	2		
Eczema	4					
Fibromyalgia		3				3
IBS	4	4	3			
Migraine	3	4	5	3	3	2
PTSD	2	3	2	3		3

BOUNDARY-INDEPENDENT CONDITIONS

DISORDER	HYPNOSIS	ACUPUNCTURE	BIOFEEDBACK	MEDITATION/ YOGA	GUIDED IMAGERY	STRESS REDUCTION
Depression	4	3	5	5	3	3
Pain*	5	4	5	4	2	3

*Note: We added the boundary-independent condition of "pain" because it commonly accompanies most of the other disorders and is also effectively treated by virtually all of the CAM approaches.

Some observers of a skeptical or cynical bent might argue that none of these CAM treatments is effective outside of the placebo effect. That is, any benefit accruing to the patient lies in her or his willingness to believe that the given approach *will* work—and thus it does. Mind over body, in other words.

There are two problems with this explanation. First, as we've seen, mind and body are not distinctly different from one another—so the assumption of "mind over body" is off base to begin with. Second (and more practically), *many people want and need a particular treatment to work for them but find, disappointingly, that it does not.* If the placebo effect were the only explanation, then we would not encounter the common problem that a particular treatment doesn't work for a given person who strongly believes that it *will* work for them. The efficacy of these treatments, therefore, must be based on aspects of human physiology that conventional science can't yet explain. In this book, our major proposition is that boundary type figures prominently in this equation.

A THUMBNAIL REFERENCE

Because boundaries cover a spectrum from thick to thin, we present here a thumbnail reference so you can quickly see how the different CAM therapies work according to boundary type, based on all the available evidence. This spectrum is presented expressly for you as a consumer-friendly step toward personalized medicine in the twenty-first century.

THIN- - - - - - - - - - - - - - - - - - -MIDPOINT- - - - - - - - - - - - - - - -THICK

| HYPNOSIS | ACUPUNCTURE | BIOFEEDBACK | GUIDED IMAGERY | STRESS REDUCTION | MEDITATION & YOGA |

RELIEVING A MIX OF CONDITIONS

If you are dealing with some combination of thick and thin boundary conditions, then you probably have a BQ score that is not especially toward either end of the spectrum. In such cases we offer two suggestions. First, choose a therapy that shows promise in relieving the type of illness that is most problematic for you. Alternatively, you could try one of the approaches (such as acupuncture, biofeedback, or guided imagery) that may be useful in alleviating *both* thick and thin boundary conditions.

A PRIMER ON CAM

Now that you know which treatments are likely to be right for you, it's a reasonable and safe bet to go ahead and try them out. Bear in mind that standard medical approaches—chiefly drugs and surgery—are not always successful themselves and, in any event, are riskier than any of the Super Seven approaches evaluated here.

The balance of this chapter offers some useful insight into the Super Seven. First, though, a word about complementary and alternative medicine itself. CAM includes what is known as "mind-body medicine," as well as healing traditions from other cultures such as acupuncture and yoga. Distinct from conventional practices that treat a given symptom or set of symptoms, CAM approaches proceed from a holistic perspective that considers the *patient* as uppermost. A link between the person's mind and body is assumed.

As we gathered earlier in this book, that view is being increasingly validated through the findings of psychoneuroimmunology, which show beyond a reasonable doubt that our immune system, our hormonal system, and our nervous system are in continuous contact. The brain and the rest of the body are two sides of the same coin. Indeed, through our enteric nervous system, we have a bona fide "mind of the gut," and, it turns out, having a gut feeling is just what we say it is. The more we learn about ourselves, the more we find we are psychosomatic beings. That's why the hyphen between *mind* and *body* should really be retired.

CAM is much closer to this unified view of human nature than is conventional medicine. The various CAM therapies, of course, emphasize different aspects of bodymind functioning. They don't constitute a single systematic theory and practice. The field is continuing to grow and change.

HYPNOSIS

Are you highly hypnotizable? About 10% of people are. Then again, about 10% of people are strongly resistant to hypnotic suggestion.[14] Everyone else is somewhere in the middle—as is the case with boundaries. In fact, extremely thin boundary people make the best hypnotic subjects because they rapidly incorporate "external" suggestions as their own.[15]

Hypnosis has been used continuously for the past 250 years. Variously known as mesmerism, animal magnetism, and magnetic healing, hypnosis has ranged from providing amusement at parties and on stage to helping people break addictions, shrink warts, and rid themselves of hives. While the actual mechanism of hypnosis is still unknown (in our previous book, we suggest it relates to breathing and blood flow[16]), verifiable changes take place in the brain and the body when someone is hypnotized.[17]

During hypnosis, a person enters a state of deep relaxation and focus while awareness of the immediate surroundings diminishes (a type of dissociation). While in this state of concentration, one becomes highly responsive to suggestion. Contrary to popular folklore, though, you cannot be hypnotized against your will. You must be willing to concentrate your thoughts and follow the suggestions offered. All forms of hypnotherapy, then, are essentially varieties of *self-hypnosis*. The process is literally brought home for many patients whose therapists provide audiotapes for them to use on their own.

Physiologically, hypnosis resembles other forms of guided relaxation. Prompted by deep breathing, it decreases activity of the sympathetic nervous system, lowering blood pressure and heart rate and generally calming our bodymind. The benefits, particularly for thin boundary conditions, can be substantial.

ACUPUNCTURE

As he worked with thin boundary people, Ernest Hartmann noted that they would often report a sense of "energy flow" in their bodies that was lacking in the observations of people with thicker boundaries.[18] Acupuncture, in particular, seems to prompt this sense of "energy moving"—a correspondence noted by scientist and author Candace Pert.[19]

An impressive amount of evidence about the benefits of acupuncture has been gathered by Western scientists since the treatment was "rediscovered" in the wake of president Nixon's 1971 visit to China. Experiments conducted in the past fifteen years, especially, have brought acupuncture much closer to mainstream acceptance. For example, the practice is known to be able to turn breech babies in utero without the costs and risks associated with typical medical interventions.[20] Indeed Mike Jawer's wife, after a single acupuncture session, felt her breech baby turn at thirty-eight weeks, enabling a safe and natural birth.

Beyond considerations of boundary type, one important reason acupuncture doesn't work for everyone is because, as practiced in the West, much of acupuncture practice is incomplete or incorrect. Part of the problem is that many forms of acupuncture recently made popular in the West are based on selected, partial, or idiosyncratic interpretations of the ancient Chinese sources. The result can be a somewhat "watered down" or simplified version that is less potent for certain people or problems.

In the same way, a remarkable depth of diagnostic information is available from those classic sources. This material is typically short-changed by Western practice, though, accustomed as it is to reducing extensive insights about the whole human being into a series of numbers, standardized tests, or biomedical procedures.

Given the demonstrated benefit of acupuncture for most thin boundary conditions, and the moderate efficacy demonstrated for several thick boundary ones, this classic bodymind practice deserves a more complete hearing. Perhaps you'll be one of those who pushes the "state of the art" forward.

BIOFEEDBACK

Biofeedback helps people to regulate various aspects of bodily functioning. By paying attention to a monitor of physiological activity, stroke patients, for example, can learn to reuse muscles in their arms or legs. Individuals who have been fitted with an artificial limb can be trained to move it as they would a real limb. Others can learn to improve bladder function. Biofeedback is also used to help people simply relax.

This form of therapy emerged in the 1960s and 1970s, when advances in psychological and medical research converged with developments in biomedical technology. By watching or listening to a monitoring device, patients could learn by trial and error to control the nervous system and other autonomic activity previously thought to be involuntary, such as blood pressure, temperature, gastrointestinal functioning, and brain wave patterns.

A major reason biofeedback is appealing is that it puts *you* in charge, giving you a sense of mastery and self-reliance over illness. This attitude can become self-reinforcing, helping reduce symptom occurrence and shorten recovery time. As noted above, biofeedback is also effective for a wide range of chronic conditions regardless of boundary type, appealing to thick boundary individuals by putting them "in charge," while benefitting thin boundary people by providing visual validation of their feelings.

MEDITATION

Over the past twenty years, meditation has changed from being predominantly a religious or spiritual practice to being used as a healthful means of relaxing and calming the bodymind. Some forms of meditation have the person focus on a single word or thought, while others emphasize attention to the breath or to a specific sound or *mantra*. All forms of meditation are aimed at stilling restless mental and emotional activity to promote quietude and calm.

Meditative practices have come to the West from a variety of cultures, especially the spiritual practices of India, China, and Japan. Meditation is also inspired by an early American tradition of deliberate, mindful experience of nature, exemplified by the New England transcendentalists. Although a contemplative, "mindful" form of meditation is popular now in the West, there are also more active forms, such as the Chinese martial art t'ai chi, the Japanese martial art aikido, and the walking meditations of Zen Buddhism.[21]

Although many Asian meditative practices have the person focus on a sound, a phrase, or a prayer in order to minimize distraction, the practice of mindfulness does the opposite. In mindfulness meditation, thoughts and feelings that arise are not ignored but observed, nonjudgmentally, as events arising in one's field of awareness. One way to envision how mindfulness works is to picture the mind as the surface of a lake or ocean. Many people think the goal of meditation is to stop the waves so that the water becomes flat, peaceful, and tranquil. In mindfulness practice, however, the aim is to simply observe the waves, moment by moment, go with the flow, and ride along.

YOGA

From its origins as a devotional or spiritual practice, yoga has become a widely popular and effective technique that emphasizes breathing and physical postures in attaining a meditative state. Its more active form, hatha yoga (physical yoga), is also popular in the West.

As with hypnosis, meditation and yoga result in a slowdown of one's metabolism, resulting in a sharp reduction in oxygen consumption and carbon dioxide output. Although blood pressure and heart rate decrease overall, peripheral blood flow increases, ensuring that oxygen is more efficiently delivered to the muscles and that lactate (a chemical that builds up with muscle fatigue) is more quickly removed. Reduction of lactate, in turn, lessens blood pressure as well as anxiety.

The relaxation induced by meditation and yoga may be deeper in some ways than that of sleep—with many attendant benefits for the bodymind. These approaches work especially well for several thick boundary conditions.

GUIDED IMAGERY

Over the last fifty years, psychologists have thoroughly examined and categorized the many types of imagery produced by the mind. The most common type of imagery, of course, is memory—what you see in your mind's eye. But imagery includes all the senses: aural (sound), tactile (touch), olfactory (smell), proprioceptive (bodily position), and kinesthetic (movement). While we tend to think of imagery as something visual, any other sense or combination of senses may be involved.

Furthermore, imagery often has a "tone" or feeling to it. This aspect of imagery is perhaps most apparent when we consider dreams, which are effectively strings of images. Some of our dreams are impressive and memorable due to the vividness of their imagery and the feelings they convey.

Through guided imagery, a person can picture (or otherwise frame) an illness or aspect of bodymind functioning—and imagine the condition changing for the better. Hypnosis and biofeedback make use of imagery as well. The practice appears helpful for several of the chronic conditions we've examined.

RELAXATION AND STRESS REDUCTION

Stress has gotten something of a bad rap. If, as Alvin Toffler postulated in his 1970 bestseller *Future Shock,*[22] people in the West at that time were being stressed to their limit, then what are we up against today? On the other hand, environmental stimulation is critically important to early childhood development as well as to survival later in life. We all need challenges, after all, to keep us on our toes. As zoologist Desmond Morris has noted, human beings' struggle is not against stressors per se but to achieve the optimum level of stimulation—not too much, not too little.[23]

Stress is not, as usually assumed, "those things out there" but instead what happens *inside the bodymind* as a person reacts. When a situation exceeds one's ability to respond or cope effectively, the stress becomes *distress*. This concept was popularized in the 1960s through the work of Dr. Hans Selye at the University of Montreal. He defined stress as the rate of wear and tear on the body—an interaction of outside stimulus and human arousal in response.[24] Some people, of course, are much quicker to become distressed than others. Their bodymind engine revs faster, leading to greater wear and tear (and illness) over time.

The pressures that encroach on our lives—workload, deadlines, traffic, crime, problems with spouses or children, job changes, relocation, and so forth—are never ending. We normally experience some degree of stress in everything we do and everything that happens to us. The key is to *learn to control our response*. This is the aim of stress management. By becoming more fully aware of how we typically respond to stressors, we can develop the ability to prevent distress.

Cardiologist Herbert Benson of Harvard Medical School is a well-known researcher into stress-reduction techniques. He identified the "relaxation response," a set of physiological and psychological benefits common to a variety of bodymind practices. These approaches all involve a quiet, calm environment, the objective of focusing the mind, a passive attitude, and a comfortable posture.[25] The chronic condition that appears to be helped the most by such systematic relaxation is hypertension, also known as high blood pressure. The word *hypertension* itself indicates the association with stress and the condition is markedly improved by stress reduction.

Exercise can also be a powerful means of reducing stress (as can laughter and sexual activity, which are themselves forms of exercise).

Regular exercise is also useful in promoting cardiovascular health, improving muscle tone, and lifting one's mood and outlook in general.

YOU HAVE THE OPTIONS

Informed by this primer—as well as your understanding of boundaries—you now have a guide to which types of treatment you might wish to use for your particular health condition (or conditions). Consult the charts toward the beginning of this chapter, consider where you are on the boundary spectrum, and select a CAM approach that holds promise for *you*.

Remember, these CAM therapies have been extensively studied over many years. They are not "off the wall" or in an early stage of development. They have helped millions of people already and saved them a substantial amount of money in the process. We are not arguing against conventional medicine, but we *are* advocating sound, safe, cost-effective treatments that—based on your boundary type—have a reasonable chance of improving your health. *These Super Seven remedies are available to help you now.*

Chapter 8

PUSHING BOUNDARIES

Treatments beyond the Super Seven

A core idea of this book has been that feelings constitute energy. As feelings stream throughout the body, so does the associated energy. An honest and forthright view of how human beings work would necessarily reflect this state of being. It makes sense, then, that all the CAM therapies we've been discussing—and still others we're going to consider—focus, to one extent or another, on the feeling body.

While it could be said that conventional medical treatments, medication and surgery foremost among them, also take feelings into account ("this procedure will make you feel better"; "this drug will reduce your pain"), their approach *imposes a solution* on the feeling body from the outside as opposed to working with it on its own terms from the inside. CAM therapies embrace the ideas that illness is a disturbance in the smooth functioning of the bodymind and, in order to restore that functioning, the doctor and patient must endeavor to help the bodymind *heal itself.*

A great deal of attention is thus given to emotions (or their corollary, feelings, that are stuck and *not* in motion) as a means of deciphering what is happening physiologically, unconsciously, and psychosomatically. CAM therapies, especially those widely regarded as forms of "energy medicine"—acupuncture, qi gong, massage, reflexology, shiatsu, reiki, therapeutic touch, and others—all presume that feelings contribute to the flow of energy a person manifests. So if the therapist can "read" and carefully adjust that flow of energy, the patient is likely to feel better.

It might be useful to recognize that the word *heal* comes from a Germanic and Old English root meaning whole or wholesome.[1] Unlike the Western medical and scientific tradition, which has sought to make people well by studying the discrete tissues, organs, and systems of the human body, Eastern traditions—mainly from China, Japan, and the Indian subcontinent—focus on the interrelationship between people and their environment, and on the signs of flow and interaction within the body. Today's complementary and alternative medicine, much of which draws heavily from Eastern sources, is thus more "wholistic" than mainstream western practice.

Wholistic (or holistic, the more popular spelling) has an appealing sound to it, as if it might be less complicated or easier to comprehend than Western medicine. But the assumptions on which Eastern practices are based are somewhat esoteric, and certainly much different than concepts we in the West have grown up with. They might strike you as strange or based on little that's "scientific." These approaches, however, are well worth learning about, if only because there is compelling evidence that they work well for many health conditions and, perhaps, even better for certain types of people.

MOVING WEST TO EAST

A key in bridging from our Western frame of reference to an Eastern understanding is recognizing that the former is concerned with structure and cause and effect, and the latter with relationship, flow, and function. Whereas Western medicine asks, "What is this? What is it made of? Where did it come from?" Eastern medicine asks, "What is its function? Into what pattern does it fit?" It was in the West that systematic studies developed, such as biology, chemistry, anatomy, and physiology, all of which detail physical form and mechanisms of action. Eastern medical approaches attend to the function something has and the larger setting where it acts. They don't ask "What x is causing y?" but rather "What is the relationship between x and y?" Thus, whereas *mainstream Western medicine tends to focus on a patient's symptoms, CAM looks first at the person experiencing them.*[2]

Eastern practices, which have sustained themselves over thousands of years, may be thought of as "prescientific" from the standpoint of Western medicine (although anthropologists view them as "ethnoscience"). However, the practices have their own internal logic and coherence. They are based on extensive clinical observations, critical thought, and testing. They originate within a culture, outlook, vocabulary, and sensibility far removed from the West. It's rather like the difference between our system of writing and the Chinese use of ideograms. This pictographic symbol—水—means water. And here is the symbol for qi—氣—which, as you may recall, suggests breath or steam. While these ideograms are vastly different from the string of letters we use to spell out words, they have no less validity.

The same holds for approaches to medicine. While Eastern medicine doesn't employ the anatomic concept of a nervous system, its "energy anatomy" and energetically based practices can be used to treat neurological disorders. It doesn't explicitly invoke the bacteria and viruses that cause pneumonia (instead using terms translated as "wind evil," or "pestilential" energy), but it can treat the disease we call pneumonia. It doesn't delineate organs or glands such as the pancreas or the adrenals, yet it does treat disorders of the pancreas and adrenal glands.[3] Indeed, because Western medicine has not yet found discrete mechanisms to explain, in its own terms, the chronic conditions addressed in this book, the Eastern concepts that underlie and inform many CAM practices are ideal to consider.[4]

QI AND THE MERIDIANS

The central concept running through Eastern healing practices (and, for that matter, the martial arts) is that of a fundamental life energy. It's known as *qi* in China (pronounced "chee"), *mana* in Polynesia, and *prana* in India. We'll refer to it from here on as qi, which can mean air, breath, or steam, but can also be translated as vitality, life force, or energy.[5] The actual pictographic symbol for qi shows steam or vapor rising over rice, which has a distinctly metabolic quality.[6]

This energy is conceptualized as universal. As it animates living things, qi is also said to surround and pervade everything (including inanimate objects), much as we in the West picture electromagnetic radiation, or even the energy-matter duality of quantum physics.

All creatures and plants constantly ingest qi as they breathe and take in nourishment. "External" qi is thus transformed into "internal" qi. Then, as the living body exhales and digests its food, the internal qi becomes "waste" qi. External qi can be healthful or harmful, just as food can. While a Western nutritionist sees vitamin-rich foods, for example, an Eastern physician would refer to foods "rich in qi." Likewise, one's internal qi can be strong enough to protect oneself from debilitating influences—either germs or stressors, as we in the West would say—or fail to protect, as the case may be. And, as alluded to earlier, suppressed or unrecognized feelings are believed to play havoc with the balance and flow of qi, reducing its strength and effectiveness.[7]

Qi is seen to flow through a system of bodily channels known as meridians. (These channels can be compared to *chakras* and *nadis* in the Hindu Ayurvedic tradition.) Disruption of the energy flow will result in disease in those parts of the body supplied by the affected meridian.[8] Chinese medicine identifies twelve pairs of meridians—the pairs corresponding to the left and right sides of the body—plus two unpaired meridians running midway through the body's front and back and six "extra" meridians comprising the links between other major meridians. Smaller channels called collaterals are also said to connect the meridians. Each of the twelve pairs of meridians is associated with an organ—so there is a lung meridian, a liver meridian, a heart meridian, and so forth. Each receives qi from another meridian and passes it on to a third meridian, so that qi circulates throughout the body much as blood circulates through the blood vessels.[9]

In fact, Chinese medicine envisions a mutually supportive relationship between qi and blood. Qi is said to give the blood vitality and direction, and the blood, in turn, is said to nourish qi by sustaining the tissues of the body. In other words, qi provides the life force, and the blood carries on its essential responsibilities, transporting food, oxygen, and fluids throughout a body fundamentally animated by qi.[10]

Eastern medicine appraises the cause of discomfort or illness based on how qi is malfunctioning or in low supply. This approach is quite different from the approach Westerners are familiar with, namely a diagnosis based on a particular disease and its effect on a given organ or part of the body. Rather than a diagnosis of, say, "uterine fibroids" or "lower back spasms," Eastern medicine presumes that the person's qi has been disrupted in such a way as to *manifest* as the functional complaints, such as pain, associated with uterine fibroids or lower back spasms. By increasing, balancing, or otherwise adjusting the flow of qi, Eastern practices aim to reverse chronic illness—a welcome departure from efforts to reduce symptoms mainly by medications or painful surgical procedures.[11]

Eastern medicine looks to the symptoms a person is experiencing for clues as to how the individual's energy is flowing and which adjustments to qi are needed. The proof of the treatment's validity lies in its *working,* even if Western science cannot explain why.[12] One suggestion is that the practices used for manipulation of qi actually boost parasympathetic activity within the autonomic nervous system, fostering the relaxation so essential to healing (see chapter 7).[13] The insertion of acupuncture needles into the skin also stimulates the release of endorphins, a potent type of endogenous painkiller. But why particular acupoints should be responsible, as mapped out millennia ago by investigators in the East, is not at all clear, nor are endorphins necessarily the correct explanation.

VITAL ENERGY: A FRESH PERSPECTIVE

In the East, qi is considered basic to human functioning. Likewise, a concept of "vital energy" or "life force" has long been an assumption of Western philosophy, but this notion was rejected in the twentieth century by Western science and medicine. Yet the idea remains planted firmly in our religion, philosophy, and literature. Hebrew, the language of the Old Testament, equates "breath" and "spirit" (remember, qi means air or breath as well as energy); the Latin word *spiritus* means "divine breath" or "inspiration"; in 1 Corinthians we read, "Do you not know that your body is a shrine of the indwelling Holy Spirit?"; Leonardo da Vinci said, "Where the spirit does not work with the hand, there is no art"; and Shakespeare wrote (in his play *Julius Caesar*), "For I am full of spirit and resolve to meet all perils very constantly." Interestingly, it has been pointed out that words, like *spirit*, beginning with "sp"—speech, spark, sprout, spit, spray, spring, even sperm—connote a "breathlike explusory act" through which something alive or active is birthed.[14] These "spirited" words are an example of the sound of the word imitating the sound of the natural phenomenon it represents (technically called *onomatopoeia*). In modern psychology, the concept of *libido* hearkens back to this age-old notion of life energy.

If we look past the divide between East and West, we can easily recognize that all human beings are organically the same. At the root of being is our capacity to *feel*. We could not feel—nor do anything else that makes us human—without energy. Whether we term it spirit, qi, prana, vim, vigor, get-up-and-go, or dispositional energy, the principle appears similar. We need not look on it as anything supernatural. The energy produced in our cells animates our bodymind. Our "spirits" are bound up with our sensations—something Chinese philosophy has long understood.[15] Not only does the quality and quantity of our bodymind energy, its ebb and flow, relate to our personality, it cannot help but influence our health at any given time.

HOW COULD ENERGY MEDICINE WORK?

We might grant that a fine needle, inserted into one of hundreds of acupoints in the body, would liberate or moderate a flow of energy. But what of other forms of energy medicine in which the activity is simply "hands on"? Acupressure, for example—which stems from the same tradition as acupuncture—relies on a person exerting pressure on the acupoints. Shiatsu (a Japanese practice in which *tsubos* are seen to function as the equivalent of acupoints), reflexology, and various forms of massage and bodywork also revolve around touch. Other bodywork practices (such as the Alexander technique, Rolfing, osteopathy, and chiropractic care) focus on adjusting relations among the bones and muscles. Still other therapies such as qi gong, reiki, and therapeutic touch don't even require that a person *be* touched. Aside from the placebo effect, wherein approximately one out of three people benefits from a drug or therapy because he or she expects to, how could such forms of energy medicine lead to healing?[16]

This question may be answered in two ways. First, by recognizing the "stealth" power that touch wields in our lives, and second, by considering that our bodymind energy does not stop within the envelope of the skin. Let's start with something we *can* grasp quickly enough: the power of touch.

TOUCH: IT'S FUNDAMENTAL

The sense of touch dominates our lives, though it's so much a part of us that we hardly realize it. Our speech illuminates its importance, though. We can't help but say things like:

I'm touched.	He can't take the pressure.
Get a grip.	Be tactful, not heavy handed.
He's cold; she's hot.	You're hitting all the right points.
That news is hard to handle.	Be firm; toe the line.
Here's my contact information.	Don't get turned around.
They're tied up right now.	Where do you stand?
Let's keep it at arm's length.	We're making strides now.
I just feel shattered, shaken up.	He's got the common touch.
Pull yourself together.	Don't be a pushover.

Don't be a sore loser.

What a letdown.

That remark was cutting.

She's got an abrasive manner.

He's a little rough around the edges.

That movie creeped me out.

I've got cold feet.

Don't be a wet blanket; come out of your shell.

I can't put my finger on it, but it just feels right.

I feel all warm and fuzzy.

I feel ten feet tall today.

I feel stuck.

I'm down in the dumps.

What they said got under my skin.

I can feel it in my bones.

That song is so stirring, so uplifting.

Am I reaching you?

He may be thick, but she is thin-skinned.

Chin up.

You've got to unwind.

What a pain in the neck you are.

My gut tells me you're wrong.

Their idea has legs, but ours is a stretch.

That's a heavy burden to shoulder.

That's deep.

Don't be so superficial.

As mentioned briefly in chapter 2, the skin is incredibly sensitive, registering temperature, pressure, pain, humidity, a wisp of air, a jolt of electricity. It is, in fact, our body's nervous system turned outward. In the womb, it affects the development of the immune system, which interacts with everything outside that is foreign to the body. Touch has been called "the mother of the senses" since it's the first to develop in the womb.[17] Our skin can sweat, it can "crawl," it can tingle, it can blanch, it can break out, it can blush. Just as we speak of emotions as *feelings*—a barometer of our internal state and our reaction to the world around us—so, too, is our skin an interface, an emissary or source of communication between inside and out. The skin is a veritable barometer of our internal states and pressures.

Touch itself—and movement toward or away from someone—can be extremely expressive. We hold a baby or a lover tenderly (popular songs refer to one's lover as "my baby"), throw a punch in anger, throw up our hands in exasperation, or turn ourselves away in sadness, resignation, or despair. ("A rock feels no pain," observed Paul Simon, "and an island never cries.")

Given how fundamental feeling and touch are in our lives, it shouldn't be surprising that virtually any therapy that involves stroking, rubbing, or kneading the skin, or manipulating the muscles will deepen breathing, improve circulation, and reduce tension. (Sexual activity also confers these benefits, and massage therapy and sexual activity in Asian tradition can be experienced either separately or together.) The physical contact involved may also strengthen the immune system, at least for a short while.[18]

The first answer to the question we raised earlier ("How could energy medicine help a person to heal?") is, therefore, fairly simple. Many energy medicine approaches rely on person-to-person contact—and it's this "hands on," "high touch," and "personal touch" that promotes bodymind relaxation and the many benefits that go with it. However, we need to go further than this relatively commonsense understanding to explain how still other energy medicine practices might work, specifically those that don't rely primarily on physical touch.

TRANSFER OF ENERGY

A second way to look at energy medicine is to consider that bodymind energy doesn't necessarily stop at the skin. Consider that practitioners of energy medicine specialize in gathering impressions about their clients' state of health from touching them or passing their hands near them. These are known as "energetic assessments" and can be gathered quickly, upon first meeting the client or after some minutes of quietly "tuning in" to whatever the client's bodymind seems to be saying. Such impressions register in a variety of ways: as intuitions; as imagery informed by feeling; as a sense of flow or blockage, ease, or density; a vital energy deficit or overabundance; a sense of pressure or fullness; a feeling of temperature differentials; a tingling sensation; or the impression of an aura around the person, its color variation indicating the condition of that particular bodymind.[19]

Practitioners tend to view themselves as conduits for energy exchange, calling themselves "givers" or "transmitters" and their clients "receivers."[20] Those receivers will sometimes feel tremendous warmth from the givers' hands—and, when it happens, the experience is quite memorable.[21]

The above descriptions are probably more than metaphorical. Certain people may, as healers, possess an ability not only to "read" the bodymind energy of others but to direct energy where needed into the bodyminds of their clients. Consider that, throughout history, the *laying on of hands* was a primary form of healing in many cultures. It was known in ancient Persia, India, and China. In classical Greece, Hippocrates—the father of modern medicine—wrote of "the force that flows from many people's hands" and commented that "the physician must be experienced in many things, most especially in rubbing."[22] Jesus of Nazareth was renowned, among other things, for his ability to cure the lame through his abilities and intentions, which were often manifested through touch and referred to as the laying on of hands. Meanwhile, halfway around the world, the ancient Chinese were beginning their delineation of acupuncture, an enterprise that would extend two thousand years and over innumerable dynasties.[23]

Interest in the presumed energy capacity of healers continues to this day. One notable experiment, conducted in 1990, showed that at least some healers can apparently produce electrical surges from their bodies. The effect was not terribly strong (a median 8.3 volts) nor the duration long (a median 3.6 seconds), but the effect was noteworthy.[24] The well-known heart surgeon Mehmet Oz has described his interest in testing "energy healers," noting his own startling observations and some of the research he's come across and even conducted experimentally during open heart surgery.[25] Our previous book, *The Spiritual Anatomy of Emotion*, draws on an extensive research base to suggest that healers are generally thin boundary people—and that the patients who gain the most benefit from somatic therapy sessions tend to be thick boundary.[26]

If some sort of energy exchange *is* involved, it's a healer's hands that are front and center. An eloquent description of what they do has been voiced by Ilana Rubenfeld, founder of the Rubenfeld Synergy form of energy medicine. As a former music student and conductor, Rubenfeld describes her hands as "listening hands":

> Through conducting, I came to understand the complexities of listening, talking and moving simultaneously. Like music, healing involves the capacity to listen to others and hear their inner song. Hearing silence as well as sounds is part of music, so the healer learns to listen to both sounds and silences. Impulses, needs, emotions and feelings in people are expressed through sounds and silences, words and wordless movements of the body. The healer listens to all these variations and helps the client achieve harmony.[27]

"As breath is visible on a mirror," Rubenfeld says, "so energy is palpable and heard by the listening hand."[28] She and all other practitioners of energy medicine believe (as we the authors have come to believe) that what they are sensing is not just energy but *energy congruent with feeling*. Whether thin boundary or thick boundary, a person's bodymind constitutes an encoded and embodied history of her or his trials and tribulations, successes and failures, heartaches and disappointments, hopes and elations. The energy "knots" or blockages seem to relate to a situation we addressed in earlier chapters of this book—namely, areas where dissociated, suppressed, or unacknowledged energy has "pooled" or been dammed up. Mainstream medicine is coming to understand that holding in our feelings has definite physical consequences.[29] But, if we envision feelings as water and their course as a stream or channel through the bodymind, we have a way to picture something that energy healers presumably *know*—that our most intense or meaningful experiences literally remain part of who we are.

Further indication of the energetics underlying human beings comes from dreaming. It's generally recognized that dreams are, in large part, about emotion—about the mind going through the day's events and classifying, remembering, or discarding them based on how they fit with previous emotionally flavored experiences.[30] Interestingly, people who have had some form of bodywork that seemed successful in getting vital energy unlocked or moving often report having powerful dreams afterward.[31] This reflects a palpable change in their bodymind state, a shift in the feeling landscape.

A REMAINING QUESTION

In this book, we've proposed that personality, as distinguished by boundary type, has a direct bearing on health. We've mentioned the hypothalamic-pituitary-adrenal (HPA) axis—the bodymind's stress-handling system—and how your stress reactivity threshold is set by genetics as well as early life experience. We've discussed how your characteristic way of handling strong feelings sets the stage for a variety of chronic conditions, from migraine, fibromyalgia, and chronic fatigue to hypertension, ulcer, and phantom pain. And now we've proposed that bodymind (or dispositional) energy, emanating from every cell of the body and intimately tied to feeling, is the reason that a variety of Eastern and energy medicine practices are therapeutic.

In all of this, we've tried to bridge the divide between Western and Eastern outlooks, attitudes, and presumptions regarding health and healing. There's another door still to open, however—a passageway of insight into an issue relevant to anyone concerned about health and human development. Namely, how is it that something as fluid as feeling can become bound up with our physicality and the types of illnesses that may become manifest later in life? Put another way: why does one thin boundary person develop irritable bowel syndrome and another, asthma? Why does one thick boundary person develop hypertension and another, chronic fatigue syndrome? Is there any rhyme or reason to the way suppressed or dissociated feelings play themselves out in the life of a human being?

There is—although it's not yet considered in the realm of medical science or reflected in standard texts on infant and child development.

The answer relates to the energy of feeling and how it "roots" itself in our bones, muscles, tendons, nerves, organs, and fascia (connecting fibers). Once again, the answer will invoke both nature and nurture.

THE INFANT'S RESPONSE TO THE WORLD

Imagine, for a moment, what it must be like for an infant before she or he understands spoken language. Undoubtedly the language of touch is primary. Gestures, facial expressions, eye contact, and tones of voice are also likely to be understood. (Think of the singsong voice most everyone adopts in speaking to babies.) And, in expressing themselves, movement and voice will be paramount for the developing infant. The baby will reach, stretch, push, contort, pull back, squeal, giggle, and cry out in pleasure, pain, and all sorts of combinations in between. All of the motor skills involved in that communication are setting a precedent, laying down a pattern, setting the stage for future expressiveness. Just as characteristic ways of thinking are being forged, so are characteristic ways of feeling.

Undoubtedly feeling is way ahead of thinking in this early period. *Comfortable*, for example, is not understood as a concept or in words; neither is *safe, warm, fearful, angry, hungry, tired, sated, frustrated, bored,* or dozens of other sensations, desires, and feelings. Infants know their *felt sense*, a term put forward by philosopher Eugene Gendlin to describe the totality of an individual's feelings at any given moment.[32]

And this process begins well before infancy. In the womb, sensory capabilities come online and the fetus is affected in myriad ways—physically by its mother's diet, health habits, and exercise, and emotionally by her stresses, cares, and upsets. Science is documenting these influences ever more keenly.[33]

In any case, the infant's emotional experience is profound because, unlike older children or adults, the baby's feelings are relatively new. If not attended to properly, these feelings can also become overwhelming—or, alternatively, a disappointment for the little person feeling them. This is why caregivers are so important. They not only react to what the infant is meaning to convey, but they *model emotional behavior* as well. And this is where things begin to get interesting.

Consider some of the ways that parents or other caregivers could misread or fail to respond to what an infant is "saying." The adults in the picture could be ambivalent about the baby in the first place. They could be preoccupied. Both parents could be at work all day. They could be depressed. They could be short-tempered. They could be uncomfortable with their own feelings or (as we saw in chapter 5 with people who are alexithymic) heedless of feelings in general.[34] They could be "magnifiers" or "globalizers," overreacting and overemphasizing relatively minor emotional signals. Or they could be inconsistent—responsive and loving in one instance and seemingly uncaring or obtuse in the next.

Through all these interactions, the infant is learning a great deal. Ultimately, he or she will learn words to identify the feelings experienced first and foremost in his or her own body: happy, sad, hurt, mad, lonely, excited, and so on. But, along the way, the developing person will learn something far more important—how to channel those feelings, how to express them or keep them at bay. The feeling stream will begin to flow in characteristic ways. To some extent, the infant will mirror or identify with what his or her caretakers appear to be feeling themselves. In other cases, the infant will gather that it's not acceptable (or, indeed, that it's counterproductive) to fully express a given emotion.[35] Compromises will be made, shortcuts taken. The stream will meander; the water will stagnate in some spots; in other places it will speed up and threaten to overrun the banks.

This process is clearly energetic. If we regard our bodymind energy as qi, the characteristic flow along the meridians has already begun to be established during infancy, or even in the womb. But, just as Chinese medicine regards qi and blood as having a reciprocal relationship, so the feeling flow becomes established materially in the body's muscles, joints, tendons, nerves, organs, and fascia. Characteristic modes of breathing, of blood flow, of posture, of unconscious defenses, and of experiencing the felt sense (or not) become entrenched. The autonomic nervous system, the endocrine system, and the immune system are all put into gear. The HPA axis acquires a set point. Our very selves become *psychosomatically real*.[36]

This is how one's personality literally takes shape. In infancy and childhood, each of us inevitably forms (or fails to adequately form)

- a sense of boundaries between oneself and others;
- a level of sensitivity to internal and external stimuli;
- an understanding of how far expressive action can be taken;
- a sense of the experiences and feelings that can be kept to oneself vs. being shared with others;
- a characteristic level of comfort or discomfort in the environment;
- a characteristic metabolic rate and stress activation set point; and
- a characteristic approach to harboring or seeking energy and excitement.[37]

In this same way, the child will develop his or her susceptibility in later life to allergies and asthma, to migraine, ulcers, rashes, chronic pain or fatigue, depression, and PTSD; in short, to all the chronic health conditions that we've examined in this book. *They all stem from the way the energy of feelings takes root in the material of the bodymind.* They are a patterned outgrowth of nascent, preverbal experience.[38]

One additional—and undoubtedly crucial—factor pertains to timing. When the child is ready to engage in a given behavior or to assert a given feeling, how do the caregivers respond? Are the feelings and behaviors encouraged and actualized, or hindered and denied? Just as there are normal physical milestones such as sitting up, crawling, walking, and talking, so all children should be ready, by a given juncture, to

- know they have a right to exist and have their core needs satisfied;
- begin to explore the world on their own;
- understand they can "make things happen" by themselves;
- integrate and express feelings of love and affection;
- form and express their opinion;
- understand the feelings and needs of others;
- recognize that some feelings can be shared and others kept to; oneself
- express and channel competitive impulses; and
- translate skills into achievement.[39]

Depending on when and how these developmental tasks are negotiated, one person's bodymind will crystallize differently than another's— *as will one's susceptibility to various chronic illnesses.*

TWO KINDS OF BODYMIND MAPS

Both West and East have ways of charting this evolution of bodymind. While these are very different, you'll also notice an overall similarity. The color diagram at the back of the book (figure 1) is produced by a school of body psychotherapists concerned with muscle tone in the clients they see.[40] "Hyporesponsive" muscles (colored blue), in their view, indicate expressive impulses that the person profiled here never developed sufficiently. The darker the blue, the less that person consciously feels muscle function in that part of the body. When prompted to take an action using that muscle, the individual is likely to say "I can't," "It's too hard," "It's too scary," and so on. (Hyporesponsiveness is akin to having a thick boundary.)

Let's say the middle part of the deltoid muscle—used by infants to raise their arm and point—as in "What's that?"—is deadened. The inference would be that, as a young child, this person was discouraged from pointing out new areas or new things to explore. Now, this particular adult is probably not one to "take what's mine" or even "point out" what's on his or her mind. We'd probably use terms such as *passive, gentle,* or *resigned* to describe this personality.

In contrast, the dark red areas in figure 1 indicate "hyperresponsive" muscles—those that show signs of overexertion and overcontrol. Suppose this person's tricep muscles (on the back of the upper arm), when tested, seem to be harder or more rigid than normal. This would denote someone who, early in life, engaged a great deal in "pushing off," in keeping people or things "at arm's length." This person might, fundamentally, be anxious about being overwhelmed or having insufficient control. (Hyperresponsiveness is akin to having a thin boundary.) We'd probably use terms such as *nervous, intense,* or *hard-driving* to describe this personality.

The green areas on the bodymap indicate flexible, resilient muscles that are neither hypo- nor hyperresponsive. The person has a normal feeling in those muscles and a fully conscious awareness of them.

The second diagram at the back of the book (figure 2) shows the principal acupuncture meridians and acupoints. The presumption here is that, when pressed or when a fine needle is inserted into them, the energy flowing through these locations will be freed up, balanced, or redirected. While figure 2 reflects an Eastern perspective and figure 1 a predominantly Western view, we can see that the aim in both cases is to better understand—wholistically—the way our bodymind functions.

TRAUMA AND HEALING

By now, you'll no doubt recognize the validity of this statement by Ilana Rubenfeld:

> Our bodies and brains house all of life's experiences. We may not be able to remember them, but they are imprinted in our unconscious. They are there, as much a part of us as our bones, heart, and bloodstream. And, whether they're pleasurable or traumatic, dramatic or insignificant, they become part of our character forever.[41]

The traumatic experiences, though, seem to register more deeply, perhaps because they contribute to survival. You undoubtedly remember where you were on that glorious late-summer morning that turned so tragic on September 11, 2001. Our bodymind ensures that the more startling, the more vividly felt an experience, the clearer the memory.

There's ample evidence, moreover, that the imprint is more resounding in some people than in others.[42] A gene has even been found that sharpens the recall of emotionally charged events.[43] The flip side is that some people are genetically primed to *forget* a traumatic event.[44] Simply put, this is the difference between thin and thick boundaries.

Heredity, though, is never the entire story. In chapter 4, we noted the relationship many researchers have found between childhood abuse and conditions such as irritable bowel syndrome, chronic fatigue, fibromyalgia, and PTSD. One could surmise, then, that "rough handling"—and, critically, one's felt reaction to it—makes a person susceptible to those ills later in life. There's even some evidence that *touch deprivation* in childhood may play a role in the development of other chronic conditions, including asthma and eczema.[45]

With a deeply ingrained experience such as trauma, traditional talk therapies are unlikely to help much. Why should they, since any event that triggered "speechless terror" (as PTSD does) is by definition beyond talk?[46] The Super Seven remedies, which are primarily experiential rather than verbal or medicinal, appear well suited for this problem. So are massage and other forms of bodywork, as well as some energy medicine practices (e.g., acupuncture and therapeutic touch).[47]

For the thick boundary person, energy medicine has shown some success in alleviating the trauma-driven symptoms of phantom pain.[48] All these approaches gently aim to help the patient access, work through, and ultimately discharge the energy that has effectively locked the trauma within his or her bodymind.

THE VALUE OF YOUR STORY

In the final analysis, any chronic illness is far more than the sum of its symptoms. Not only do certain health conditions relate to one's personality type, but understood correctly, they shed light on the intricate workings of our bodymind and the development of each person as a unique individual.

Bodyworker Deane Juhan makes the case eloquently:

> When all is well with [our body], it simply does for us, delivering the goods and paying the bills, administering our desires without troubling us with all of the pedestrian, functional details. And while this is certainly in some ways an ideal to be wished for, it is not the way that we learn certain things about ourselves.
>
> Our pains announce deficiencies, excesses, breakages, displacements, shifting balances within the complexities of our organic lives, and often in order to resolve them we have to learn something about these complicated internal affairs of ours, their rich interconnectedness, their crucial interdependencies . . . Herein is the spur for a great deal of human progress, and for that particularly potent satisfaction of having found a way out of the maze, or discovering a solution to the problem. For this experience of self-examination and revelation, we *require* situations that the experts cannot resolve, situations which throw us back onto our own resources. This is how we learn that we *have* resources.[49]

This book has aimed to give you the resources—to take your health into your own hands. Through the concept of boundaries, you now have the means to seek out cost-effective and noninvasive medical approaches that are right for *you*. You also have a greater appreciation for the bodymind basis of personality than do most physicians, psychologists, and human development experts.

To truly heal—to gain liberation from the chronic ailments we have examined—one must reclaim one's dissociated, bodily anchored feelings. That means transcending the patterns of the past. You must open yourself up to e-motion that has been neglected, held back, ignored, or suppressed. "The longer I am sick," wrote Kat Duff, a chronic fatigue sufferer, "the more I realize that illness is to health what dreams are to waking life—the reminder of what is forgotten, the bigger picture working toward resolution."[50] Incisively, she notes that "illness is not just something that happens to us, like a sudden sneeze or passing storm; it is part of who we are all the time."[51]

Not all sickness is like that. Some diseases, some infections, are fickle. They just happen, leaving us wounded and wondering in their wake. But the Dozen Discomforts we've looked at hearken back to a much earlier period in a person's life and the characteristic way he or she handled stressful circumstances and strong, difficult feelings. With each of these boundary conditions, the dissociated energy of feeling lives on in the person's bodymind—or else the pattern of dissociation continues into the present.

These stubborn patterns hold the key to your health. As the alchemists of old and the homeopaths of today have maintained, the cure can be extracted from the disease.[52] Many indigenous healers have long recognized the body's wisdom. In their traditions, psychosomatic disorders are understood to have a meaning. The goal is not simply to overcome or eliminate the symptoms but to try to see them in the context of the whole person.[53] This approach differs markedly from—indeed, it's almost the opposite of—today's standard model, geared as it is to remove or medicate the symptoms overtly causing trouble and treating the suffering person almost as an afterthought.

By realizing your boundary type, you will come home to yourself. Your story remains to be written, and your life energy is your birthright. Use the challenges posed by your chronic illness as a way to go deeper into yourself, to discover—in the words of poet Rainer Maria Rilke—"how deep the place is from which your life flows."[54]

THE BOUNDARY QUESTIONNAIRE

Below is the full-length Boundary Questionnaire developed by Dr. Ernest Hartmann. Afterward is a key for you to score your responses.

Note: While the statements are phrased in a general way, none of them is meant as a value judgment. There are no right or wrong responses. Consider these statements merely as prompts intended to sound you out on where you are right now in your life.

That being said, please rate each of the following statements from 0 to 4. A rating of 0 indicates "not at all" or "not at all true of me," whereas a rating of 4 indicates "yes, definitely" or "very true of me." Try to respond to all of the statements as quickly as you can.

1. When I wake up in the morning, I am not sure whether I am really awake for a few minutes. 0 1 2 3 4

2. I have had unusual reactions to alcohol. 0 1 2 3 4

3. My feelings blend into one another. 0 1 2 3 4

4. I am very close to my childhood feelings. 0 1 2 3 4

5. I am very careful about what I say to people until I get to know them really well. 0 1 2 3 4

6. I am very sensitive to other people's feelings.　　0 1 2 3 4

7. I like to pigeonhole things as much as possible.　　0 1 2 3 4

8. I like solid music with a definite beat.　　0 1 2 3 4

9. I think children have a special sense of joy and wonder that is later often lost.　　0 1 2 3 4

10. In an organization, everyone should have a definite place and a specific role.　　0 1 2 3 4

11. People of different nations are basically very much alike.　　0 1 2 3 4

12. There are a great many forces influencing us that science does not understand at all.　　0 1 2 3 4

13. I have dreams, daydreams, or nightmares in which my body or someone else's body is being stabbed, injured, or torn apart.　　0 1 2 3 4

14. I have had unusual reactions to marijuana.　　0 1 2 3 4

15. Sometimes I don't know whether I am thinking or feeling.　　0 1 2 3 4

16. I can remember things from when I was less than three years old.　　0 1 2 3 4

17. I expect other people to keep a certain distance.　　0 1 2 3 4

18. I think I would be a good psychotherapist.　　0 1 2 3 4

19. I keep my desk and worktable neat and well organized.　　0 1 2 3 4

20. I think it might be fun to wear medieval armor.　　0 1 2 3 4

21. A good teacher needs to help a child remain special.　　0 1 2 3 4

22. When making a decision, you shouldn't let your feelings get in the way.　　0 1 2 3 4

23. Being dressed neatly and cleanly is very important.　　0 1 2 3 4

24. There is time for thinking and there is a time for feeling; they should be kept separate.　　0 1 2 3 4

25. My daydreams don't always stay in control.　　0 1 2 3 4

26. I have had unusual reactions to coffee or tea.   0 1 2 3 4

27. For me, things are black or white; there are no shades
    of gray.   0 1 2 3 4

28. I had a difficult and complicated childhood.   0 1 2 3 4

29. When I get involved with someone, I know exactly
    who I am and who the other person is. We may   0 1 2 3 4
    cooperate, but we maintain our separate selves.

30. I am easily hurt.   0 1 2 3 4

31. I get to appointments right on time.   0 1 2 3 4

32. I like heavy, solid clothing.   0 1 2 3 4

33. Children and adults have a lot in common. They
    should give themselves a chance to be together   0 1 2 3 4
    without any strict roles.

34. In getting along with other people in an organization,
    it is very important to be flexible and adaptable.   0 1 2 3 4

35. I believe many of the world's problems could be
    solved if only people trusted each other more.   0 1 2 3 4

36. Either you are telling the truth or you are lying; that's
    all there is to it.   0 1 2 3 4

37. I spend a lot of time daydreaming, fantasizing, or in
    reverie.   0 1 2 3 4

38. I am afraid I may fall apart completely.   0 1 2 3 4

39. I like to have beautiful experiences without analyzing
    them or trying to understand them in detail.   0 1 2 3 4

40. I have definite plans for my future. I can lay out pretty
    well what I expect year by year at least for the next   0 1 2 3 4
    few years.

41. I can usually tell what another person is thinking or
    feeling without anyone saying anything.   0 1 2 3 4

42. I am unusually sensitive to loud noises and to bright
    lights.   0 1 2 3 4

43. I am good at keeping accounts and keeping track of my money.   0 1 2 3 4

44. I like stories that have a definite beginning, middle, and end.   0 1 2 3 4

45. I think an artist must in part remain a child.   0 1 2 3 4

46. A good organization is one in which all the lines of responsibility are precise and clearly established.   0 1 2 3 4

47. Each nation should be clear about its interests and its boundaries, as well as the interests and boundaries of other nations.   0 1 2 3 4

48. There is a place for everything, and everything should be in its place.   0 1 2 3 4

49. Every time something frightening happens to me, I have nightmares, fantasies, or flashbacks involving the frightening event.   0 1 2 3 4

50. I feel unsure of who I am at times.   0 1 2 3 4

51. At times I feel happy and sad all at once.   0 1 2 3 4

52. I have a clear memory of my past. I could tell you pretty well what happened year by year.   0 1 2 3 4

53. When I get involved with someone, we sometimes get too close.   0 1 2 3 4

54. I am a very sensitive person.   0 1 2 3 4

55. I like things to be spelled out precisely and specifically.   0 1 2 3 4

56. I think a good teacher must remain in part a child.   0 1 2 3 4

57. I like paintings and drawings with clear outlines and no blurred edges.   0 1 2 3 4

58. A good relationship is one in which everything is clearly defined and spelled out.   0 1 2 3 4

59. People are totally different from each other.   0 1 2 3 4

60. When I wake up, I wake up quickly and am absolutely sure I am awake.   0 1 2 3 4

61. At times I have felt as if I were coming apart. 0 1 2 3 4

62. My thoughts blend into one another. 0 1 2 3 4

63. I had a difficult and complicated adolescence. 0 1 2 3 4

64. Sometimes it's scary when one gets too involved with another person. 0 1 2 3 4

65. I enjoy soaking up atmosphere even if I don't understand exactly what's going on. 0 1 2 3 4

67.*I like paintings or drawings with soft and blurred edges. 0 1 2 3 4

68. A good parent has to be a bit of a child too. 0 1 2 3 4

69. I cannot imagine marrying or living with someone of another religion. 0 1 2 3 4

70. It is very hard truly to empathize with another person because people are so different. 0 1 2 3 4

71. All important thought involves feelings too. 0 1 2 3 4

72. I have dreams, daydreams, or nightmares in which I see isolated body parts—arms, legs, heads, and so on. 0 1 2 3 4

73. Things around me seem to change their size and shape. 0 1 2 3 4

74. I can easily imagine myself to be an animal or what it might be like to be an animal. 0 1 2 3 4

75. I feel very separate and distinct from everyone else. 0 1 2 3 4

76. When I am in a new situation, I try to find out precisely what is going on and what the rules are as soon as possible. 0 1 2 3 4

77. I enjoy(ed) geometry; there are simple, straightforward rules and everything fits. 0 1 2 3 4

---

*There was no question 66 on Dr. Hartmann's original Boundary Questionnaire, but no worries—it's an old oversight from his early work and he and his colleagues have worked around it. Nothing is actually omitted.

78. A good parent must be able to empathize with his or her children, and to be their friend and playmate at the same time.　　0 1 2 3 4

79. I cannot imagine living with or marrying a person of another race.　　0 1 2 3 4

80. People are so different that I never know what someone else is thinking or feeling.　　0 1 2 3 4

81. Beauty is a very subjective thing. I know what I like, but I wouldn't expect anyone else to agree.　　0 1 2 3 4

82. In my daydreams, people kind of merge into one another or one person turns into another.　　0 1 2 3 4

83. My body sometimes seems to change its size or shape.　　0 1 2 3 4

84. I get overinvolved in things.　　0 1 2 3 4

85. When something happens to a friend of mine or a lover, it is almost as if it happened to me.　　0 1 2 3 4

86. When I work on a project, I don't like to tie myself down to a definite outline. I rather like to let my mind wander.　　0 1 2 3 4

87. Good solid frames are very important for a picture or painting.　　0 1 2 3 4

88. I think children need strict discipline.　　0 1 2 3 4

89. People are happier with their own kind than mixing with others.　　0 1 2 3 4

90. "East is east and west is west and never the twain shall meet." (Kipling)　　0 1 2 3 4

91. There are definite rules and standards, which one can learn, about what is and is not beautiful.　　0 1 2 3 4

92. In my dreams, people sometimes merge into each other or become other people.　　0 1 2 3 4

93. I believe I am influenced by forces that no one can understand.　　0 1 2 3 4

94. When I read something, I get so involved it can be difficult to get back to reality.　　0 1 2 3 4

95. I trust people easily.　　0 1 2 3 4

96. When I am working on a project, I make a careful, detailed outline and then follow it closely.　　0 1 2 3 4

97. The movies and TV shows I like the best are the ones with good guys and bad guys, and you always know who they are.　　0 1 2 3 4

98. If we open ourselves to the world, we find that things go better than expected.　　0 1 2 3 4

99. Most people are sane; some people are crazy; there is no in-between.　　0 1 2 3 4

100. I have had déjà vu experiences.　　0 1 2 3 4

101. I have a very definite sense of space around me.　　0 1 2 3 4

102. When I really get involved in a game or in playing at something, it's sometimes hard when the game stops and the rest of the world begins.　　0 1 2 3 4

103. I am a very open person.　　0 1 2 3 4

104. I think I would enjoy being an engineer.　　0 1 2 3 4

105. There are no sharp dividing lines between normal people, people with problems, and people who are considered psychotic or crazy.　　0 1 2 3 4

106. When I listen to music, I get so involved it is sometimes difficult to get back to reality.　　0 1 2 3 4

107. I am always at least a little bit on my guard.　　0 1 2 3 4

108. I am a down-to-earth, no-nonsense kind of person.　　0 1 2 3 4

109. I like houses with flexible spaces, where you can shift things around and make different uses out of the same rooms.　　0 1 2 3 4

110. Success is largely a matter of good organization and keeping good records.　　0 1 2 3 4

111. Everyone is a little crazy at times.   0 1 2 3 4

112. I have daymares.   0 1 2 3 4

113. I awake from one dream into another.   0 1 2 3 4

114. Time slows down and speeds up for me. Time passes
     very differently on different occasions.   0 1 2 3 4

115. I feel at one with the world.   0 1 2 3 4

116. Sometimes I meet someone and trust him or her so
     completely that I can share just about everything   0 1 2 3 4
     about myself at the first meeting.

117. I think I would enjoy being the captain of a ship.   0 1 2 3 4

118. Good fences make good neighbors.   0 1 2 3 4

119. My dreams are so vivid that even later I can't tell them
     from waking reality.   0 1 2 3 4

120. I have often had the experience of different senses
     coming together. For example, I have felt that I could   0 1 2 3 4
     smell a color, or see a sound, or hear an odor.

121. I read things straight through from beginning to end.
     (I don't skip or go off on interesting tangents.)   0 1 2 3 4

122. I have friends and I have enemies, and I know which
     are which.   0 1 2 3 4

123. I think I would enjoy being some kind of creative
     artist.   0 1 2 3 4

124. A man is a man and a woman is a woman; it is very
     important to maintain that distinction.   0 1 2 3 4

125. I know exactly which parts of town are safe and which
     parts are unsafe.   0 1 2 3 4

126. I have had the experience of not knowing whether I
     was imagining something or it was actually happening.   0 1 2 3 4

127. When I recall a conversation or a piece of music, I hear
     it just as though it was happening there again right in   0 1 2 3 4
     front of me.

128. I think I would enjoy a really loose, flexible job where I could write my own job description.　0 1 2 3 4

129. All men have something feminine in them, and all women have something masculine in them.　0 1 2 3 4

130. In my dreams, I have been a person of the opposite sex.　0 1 2 3 4

131. I have had the experience of someone calling me or speaking my name, and not being sure whether it was really happening or whether I was imagining it.　0 1 2 3 4

132. I can visualize something so vividly that it is just as though it is happening right in front of me.　0 1 2 3 4

133. I think I could be a good fortune teller or a medium.　0 1 2 3 4

134. In my dreams, I am always myself.　0 1 2 3 4

135. I see auras or fields of energy around people.　0 1 2 3 4

136. I can easily imagine myself to be someone of the opposite sex.　0 1 2 3 4

137. I like clear, precise borders.　0 1 2 3 4

138. I have had the feeling that someone who is close to me was in danger or was hurt, although I had no ordinary way of knowing it, and later found out that it was true.　0 1 2 3 4

139. I have a very clear and distinct sense of time.　0 1 2 3 4

140. I like houses where rooms have definite walls and each room has a definite function.　0 1 2 3 4

141. I have had dreams that later came true.　0 1 2 3 4

142. I like fuzzy borders.　0 1 2 3 4

143. I have had "out of body" experiences during which my mind seemed to, or actually did, leave my body.　0 1 2 3 4

144. I like straight lines.　0 1 2 3 4

145. I like wavy or curved lines better than I like straight lines.　0 1 2 3 4

146. I feel sure that I can empathize with the very old.　0 1 2 3 4

SCORING THE BOUNDARY QUESTIONNAIRE

A score sheet is presented below. All the statements listed in the left-hand column are "thin" items; the statements in the right-hand column are "thick" items. The differences should be clear from reading the items.

Under each number in the left-hand column, enter the response you circled for that item. Under each number in the right-hand column, enter the *inverse* of your response, according to the following table:

4 = 0   3 = 1   2 = 2   1 = 3   0 = 4

Add the scores entered in both columns to obtain your total for each of the twelve themed categories plus your overall total at the bottom of the score sheet. (On the average, the total for all questions is 250–300.)

It's worth mentioning that one can be a thin or thick boundary person overall and yet have a different type of boundary score within the various categories. No one is reducible to a single location on the boundary spectrum. Each of us is likely to be thin in some respects, thick in others.

BOUNDARY QUESTIONNAIRE SCORE SHEET

	THIN ITEMS Score by adding what you circled from 0–4 for the given question numbers.	THICK ITEMS Score by adding the inverse of what you circled for the given question numbers.	SCORE
Category 1: Sleeping/waking/ dreaming	1, 13, 25, 37, 49, 72, 82, 92, 112, 113, 119, 130	60, 134	_____
Category 2: Unusual experiences	2, 14, 26, 38, 50, 61, 73, 83, 93, 100, 114, 120, 126, 131, 135, 138, 141, 143	(101, though not actually included in the score.)	_____
Category 3: Thoughts/feelings/ moods	3, 15, 39, 51, 62, 74, 84, 94, 102, 106, 115, 127, 132, 136	27, 139	_____

	THIN ITEMS Score by adding what you circled from 0–4 for the given question numbers.	THICK ITEMS Score by adding the inverse of what you circled for the given question numbers.	SCORE
Category 4: Childhood/ adolescence/ adulthood	4, 16, 28, 63	40, 52	_____
Category 5: Interpersonal	41, 53, 64, 85, 95, 103, 116, 146	5, 29, 122, 125 (Also: 17, 75, and 107, though not actually included in the score.)	_____
Category 6: Sensitivity	6, 18, 30, 42, 54	no items	_____
Category 7: Neatness/exactness/ precision	65, 86	7, 19, 31, 43, 55, 76, 96, 108, 121	_____
Category 8: Edges/lines/clothing	67, 109, 123, 128, 133, 142, 145	44, 57, 77, 87, 97, 104, 117, 137, 140, 144 (Also: 8, 20, and 32, though not included in the score.)	_____
Category 9: Opinions about children and others	9, 21, 33, 45, 56, 68, 78	88	_____
Category 10: Opinions about organizations and relationships	34, 98	10, 22, 46, 58, 69, 79, 89, 110	_____
Category 11: Opinions about peoples, nations, and groups	11, 35, 105, 111, 129	23, 47, 59, 70, 80, 90, 99, 118, 124	_____
Category 12: Opinions about beauty and truth	12, 71, 81	24, 36, 48, 91	_____

THICK BOUNDARY----------------------**MIDDLE**--------------------------**THIN BOUNDARY**

| 0 | 50 | 100 | 150 | 200 | 250 | 300 | 350 | 400 | 450 | 500 | 550 | 580 |

SELECTED STUDIES

Supporting the Effectiveness of CAM Treatments for the Dozen Discomforts

The findings presented in chapter 7 regarding the efficacy of the Super Seven remedies for a variety of chronic conditions are drawn from Dr. Marc Micozzi's twenty years of experience compiling and reviewing thousands of studies for his textbook, *Fundamentals of Complementary and Alternative Medicine*. Now in its fourth edition, this text is considered the standard reference for physicians and scientists practicing and researching complementary and alternative medicine. A short sample of the studies covered—as well as related research—is presented through the cross-section below.

ACUPUNCTURE

A study undertaken by a German researcher, Antonius Schneider, found that, contrary to expectation, patients with high "perceived body sensation" (a rough equivalent of thin boundaries) had a poor treatment response to acupuncture, whereas patients with low perceived body sensation (a rough equivalent of thick boundaries) had a good treatment response. "Treatment response" refers to patients' reaction to prophylactic acupuncture for postoperative nausea and vomiting.[1]

BIOFEEDBACK

In one study, thirty patients with fibromyalgia received biofeedback and experienced statistically significant improvements in mental clarity, mood, and sleep.[2]

Biofeedback techniques have also been used successfully to treat problems such as insomnia, chronic fatigue, and body pain. While biofeedback was not shown to be superior to standard care, patients who received biofeedback had significantly improved scores for hospital anxiety and depression.[3]

Nearly one hundred patients with the rheumatoid condition of systemic lupus were assigned randomly to receive biofeedback-assisted treatment or usual medical care. Those who received biofeedback had significantly greater reductions in pain and psychological functioning over controls. At a nine-month follow-up, the biofeedback group continued to exhibit relative benefit compared with controls.[4]

The Department of Psychiatry at Robert Wood Johnson Medical School in New Jersey evaluated the effectiveness of biofeedback as a complementary treatment for nearly one hundred patients with asthma. Compared with the two control groups (placebo and wait list), subjects in the two biofeedback groups were prescribed less medication, showing biofeedback to be a useful adjunct to asthma treatment that may help to reduce dependence on steroid medications.[5]

HYPNOSIS

One of the most dramatic early uses of hypnosis was for skin disorders. In the mid-1950s, anesthesiologist Arthur Mason used hypnosis to effectively treat a sixteen-year-old patient who had warts. Within ten days the warts fell off and were replaced by normal skin.[6] Since that time, hypnosis has been used to dramatically improve other skin disorders.[7]

Hypnotherapy may also have direct clinical effects on certain chronic diseases, such as reduction of bleeding in hemophiliac patients, stabilization of blood sugar in diabetic patients, and reduction in the severity of asthma attacks.[8]

Ran Anbar, a pediatric pulmonologist at State University of New York's Upstate Medical University in Syracuse, teaches children self-hypnosis to help them control their allergies and asthma.[9]

For many years, Wendy Gonsalkorale has been researching the benefits of hypnotherapy for irritable bowel syndrome at University Hospital of South Manchester (United Kingdom). In only three months, symptoms such as pain and bloating, as well as the level of "disease interference" with life, changed profoundly for most of the 232 participants.[10]

Gonsalkorale has also found good evidence for hypnotherapy's benefit to IBS patients for up to six years following treatment. In over two hundred patients, of the 71% who responded to hypnotherapy, 81% maintained their improvement, and the remaining 19% claimed that deterioration of symptoms had been slight.[11] The efficacy of hypnosis to treat irritable bowel syndrome is also extensively documented by researchers working in the United States, the United Kingdom, and elsewhere.[12]

Many controlled studies have demonstrated that hypnosis is an effective way to reduce migraine attacks in children and teenagers. In one experiment, thirty schoolchildren were either randomly assigned a placebo, given the drug propranolol (a blood pressure–lowering agent), or taught self-hypnosis. Only the children who used the self-hypnosis techniques had a significant decrease in the severity and frequency of headaches.[13]

GUIDED IMAGERY

Guided imagery has been found to have the capacity to dramatically affect the oxygen supply in tissues,[14] to influence cardiovascular,[15] vascular, or thermal response,[16] as well as the pupillary and cochlear reflexes,[17] heart rate, galvanic skin responses,[18] and salivation.[19]

Imagery can contribute to the remediation of physical problems, as documented extensively for chronic pain control. In one method, the individual allows an image of his or her pain to emerge. The person may create an image that characterizes the painful area, for example, then create a second image to counteract it. Once the images are formed, the person uses a relaxation or meditation technique to engage his or her self-healing capacity.[20]

Nurses at Ephrata Community Hospital in Pennsylvania found that offering their patients guided imagery compact discs can be effective in a variety of ways. They reported that guided imagery (1) helps patients relieve pain and anxiety before and after surgery, (2) helps to reduce high blood pressure, and (3) reduces the need for breathing and respiratory devices.[21]

Differences in pain control were examined at Kent State's College of Nursing, where forty-two patients were randomly assigned to treatment and control groups. Those who received guided imagery had decreased pain during the last two days of the four-day trial.[22]

MEDITATION

In 1968, Harvard's Herbert Benson was asked by the Maharishi International University to test Transcendental Meditation (TM) practitioners on their ability to lower their blood pressure. Benson's studies showed that TM was associated with reduced health care costs, increased longevity, and better quality of life.[23] Other studies subsequently showed that TM can result in reduced anxiety, reduced blood pressure, and reduced serum cholesterol levels[24]; that it represents a viable treatment for post-traumatic stress disorder in Vietnam veterans[25]; and that TM can lead to a reduction in chronic pain.[26]

In a follow-up study of 127 African American elders, it was found that both TM and progressive muscle relaxation significantly lowered blood pressure compared with controls, and that TM was significantly more effective than progressive muscle relaxation techniques.[27]

The term mindfulness was coined by Jon Kabat-Zinn, Ph.D., known for his work using mindfulness meditation to help medical patients with chronic pain and stress-related disorders.[28] The consistent practice of mindfulness meditation has been shown to decrease the subjective experience of pain and stress in a variety of research settings. One study found a 65% improvement in pain symptoms and a 60% improvement in sleep and fatigue levels in a sample of seventy-seven patients with fibromyalgia.[29]

PHANTOM PAIN

An assessment of the benefits of acupuncture, therapeutic touch, and other forms of "energy medicine" for patients afflicted by phantom pain has been carried out by Eric Leskowitz, director of the Integrative Medicine Project at Spaulding Rehabilitation Hospital in Boston.[30]

YOGA

Clinical studies demonstrate that yoga is an effective therapy for a range of chronic conditions, as well as for stress management. For example, yoga has been found helpful in the treatment of heart disease and high blood pressure.[31] Yoga is also useful in the management of asthma and other breathing disorders. Furthermore, it helps improve mood and counter mild depression.[32]

A number of musculoskeletal disorders and common occupational health problems can be managed with yoga. These include carpal tunnel syndrome, osteoarthritis, and lower back pain. Preliminary evidence indicates that yoga may also be helpful in disorders of the immune system, such as rheumatoid arthritis and lupus. Yoga and meditation have also improved academic and physical performance in schoolchildren.[33]

Sources for Further Information

It's a wide world, and numerous sources exist for specialized information on the health conditions and CAM therapies addressed in *Your Emotional Type*. As a service to readers who would like to know more, the following pages list nearly 350 pertinent organizations, including professional associations, research societies, educational foundations, advocacy groups, patient forums, and compilations of service providers.

The headings are not by boundary type but by subject matter as conventionally understood. Thus, you may find conditions listed together that we have suggested are of a different boundary type— chronic fatigue syndrome and fibromyalgia, for instance, or irritable bowel syndrome and ulcer. This is not done to confuse matters but because organizations are often grouped together that way when an Internet search is undertaken.

You'll find organizations and other resources located in the United States, Canada, and the United Kingdom, where we expect most of our readers are located. In some cases, European groups are listed.

Please note:

The resources listed are not intended to replace the advice or care of a medical doctor. The authors of *Your Emotional Type* have attempted to provide listings that are highly relevant and informative, but we (along with the book's publisher) disclaim responsibility for any liability, loss, or risk, personal or otherwise, that may be incurred as a consequence of applying the information presented by any of the websites listed.

The headings are alphabetical as follows:

Allergy/Asthma

Alternative Medicine—General

   AltMed—Ayurvedic

   AltMed—Chiropractic

   AltMed—Naturopathic

   AltMed—Orthopaedic

   AltMed—Osteopathic

Anxiety/Depression

Asian Therapies (Acupuncture, Acupressure, T'ai Chi, Qigong)

Biofeedback

Bodymind Connectedness

Chronic Fatigue Syndrome

Chronic Pain/Phantom Pain

Fibromyalgia/Rheumatoid Arthritis

Guided Imagery

Highly Sensitive (Very Thin Boundary) People

Hypertension

Hypnotherapy

Immune Disorders/ Environmental Health

Irritable Bowel Syndrome/ Ulcer

Meditation/Stress Reduction/Yoga

Migraine

Personality Research

Post-traumatic Stress Disorder

Psoriasis/Eczema

Somatic and Energy Therapies

Women's Health

ALLERGY/ASTHMA

American Academy of Allergy, Asthma and Immunology
www.aaaai.org

American College of Allergy, Asthma and Immunology
www.acaai.org

British Society for Allergy and Clinical Immunology
www.bsaci.org

Canadian Society of Allergy and Clinical Immunology
http://csaci.ca

European Academy of Allergy and Clinical Immunology
www.eaaci.net

National Society for Research into Allergy (UK)
www.all-allergy.org

World Allergy Organization
www.worldallergy.org

ALTERNATIVE MEDICINE—GENERAL

Academic Consortium for Complementary and Alternative Healthcare
www.accahc.org

Alternative Medicine Foundation
www.amfoundation.org

American Association of Integrative Medicine
www.aaimedicine.com

American Board of Holistic Medicine
www.amerboardholisticmed.org

American Holistic Health Association
www.ahha.org

American Holistic Medical Association
www.holisticmedicine.org

American Holistic Nurses Association
www.ahna.org

Arizona Center for Integrative Medicine (University of Arizona)
http://integrativemedicine.arizona.edu

British Complementary Medicine Association
www.bcma.co.uk

British Holistic Medical Association
www.bhma.org

Canadian Holistic Nurses Association
www.chna.ca

Canadian Institute of Natural and Integrative Medicine
www.cinim.org

Canadian Interdisciplinary Network for Complementary and Alternative Medicine Research
www.incomresearch.ca

Canadian Interdisciplinary Network for Complementary and Alternative Medicine Research
www.incamresearch.ca

Center for Integrative Medicine (University of Maryland)
www.compmed.umm.edu

Center for Integrative Medicine (University of Pittsburgh Medical Center)
http://integrativemedicine.upmc.com

Center for Spirituality and Healing (University of Minnesota)
www.csh.umn.edu

Complementary Therapists Association (UK and Ireland)
www.ctha.com

Consortium of Academic Health Centers for Integrative Medicine
www.imconsortium.org

Continuum Center for Health and Healing (Beth Israel Medical Center)
www.healthandhealingny.com

Council for Healing
www.councilforhealing.org

Duke Integrative Medicine (Duke University)
www.dukeintegrativemedicine.org

Federation of Holistic Therapists (UK)
www.fht.org.uk

Foundation for Alternative and Integrative Medicine
www.nfam.org

George Washington Institute for Spirituality and Health
www.gwish.org

Health Action Network Society (CAN)
www.hans.org

Institute for Complementary and Natural Medicine (UK)
www.i-c-m.org.uk

International Association of Healthcare Practitioners
www.iahp.com

International Society for Complementary Medicine Research
www.iscmr.org

Mayo Clinic Integrative Medicine
www.mayoclinic.org/general-internal-medicine-rst/cimc.html

Myrna Brind Center of Integrative Medicine (Thomas Jefferson University Hospitals)
www.jeffersonhospital.org/cim

National Center for Complementary and Alternative Medicine (National Institutes of Health)
http://nccam.nih.gov

Natural Health Practitioners of Canada
www.nhpcanada.org

Natural Healers (compendium of natural healing and massage schools)
www.naturalhealers.com

Network of Researchers in the Public Health of Complementary and Alternative Medicine
www.norphcam.org

Osher Center for Integrative Medicine (University of California— San Francisco)
www.osher.ucsf.edu

Osher Research Center (Harvard Medical School)
www.osher.hms.harvard.edu

PedCam (Pediatric CAM Research and Education Network)
www.pedcam.ca

Research Council for Complementary Medicine (UK)
www.rccm.org.uk

Samueli Institute
www.siib.org

Scripps Center for Integrative Medicine
www.scripps.org/services/integrative-medicine

UCLA Collaborative Centers for Integrative Medicine
http://ccim.med.ucla.edu

University of Michigan Integrative Medicine
www.med.umich.edu/umim

ALT MED—AYURVEDIC

Ayurvedic Practitioners Assoc. (UK)
www.apa.uk.com

National Ayurvedic Medical
Association
www.ayurveda-nama.org

ALT MED—CHIROPRACTIC

American Chiropractic Association
www.americhiro.org

Association of Chiropractic Colleges
www.chirocolleges.org

Canadian Chiropractic Association
www.chiropracticcanada.ca

Council on Chiropractic Education
www.cce-usa.org

Councils on Chiropractic Education
International
www.cceintl.org

Foundation for Chiropractic
Education and Research
www.fcer.org

International Chiropractors Assoc.
www.chiropractic.org

World Federation of Chiropractic
www.wfc.org

ALT MED—NATUROPATHIC

American Association of
Naturopathic Physicians
www.naturopathic.org

Association of Accredited
Naturopathic Medical Colleges
www.aanmc.org

Association of Physical and Natural
Therapists (UK)
www.apnt.org

Canadian Association of
Naturopathic Doctors
www.cand.ca

Council on Naturopathic Medical
Education
www.cnme.org

Naturopathic Physicians Research
Institute
http://nprinstitute.org

ALT MED—ORTHOPAEDIC

American Academy of Orthopaedic
Surgeons
www.aaos.org

American Association of
Orthopaedic Medicine
www.aaomed.org

British Orthopaedic Association
www.boa.ac.uk

British Orthopaedic Research
Society
www.borsoc.org.uk

Canadian Orthopaedic Association
www.coa-aco.org

Society of Orthopaedic Medicine
www.somed.org

ALT MED—OSTEOPATHIC

American Academy of Osteopathy
www.academyofosteopathy.org

American Association of Colleges of
Osteopathic Medicine
www.aacom.org

American Osteopathic Association
www.osteopathic.org

British Osteopathic Association
www.osteopathy.org

Canadian Osteopathic Association
www.osteopathic.ca

ANXIETY/DEPRESSION

Anxiety Disorders Association of
America
www.adaa.org

Anxiety Disorders Association of
Canada
www.anxietycanada.ca

Brain and Behavior Research Fund
www.narsad.org

Canadian Mental Health Association
www.cmha.ca

Mental Health America
www.nmha.org

Stress and Anxiety Research Society
www.star-society.org

ASIAN THERAPIES (ACUPUNCTURE, ACUPRESSURE, T'AI CHI, QIGONG)

Acupuncture Foundation of Canada
Institute
www.afcinstitute.com

American Academy of Medical
Acupuncture
www.medicalacupuncture.org

American Association of Oriental
Medicine
www.aaom.org

American Organization for
Bodywork Therapies of Asia
www.aobta.org

American Tai Chi and Qigong
Association
www.americantaichi.org

British Acupuncture Council
www.acpuncture.org.uk

British Medical Acupuncture Society
www.medical-acupuncture.co.uk

Canadian Association of
Acupuncture and Traditional
Chinese Medicine
www.caatcm.com

Chinese Medicine and Acupuncture
Association of Canada
www.cmaac.ca

Council of Colleges of Acupuncture
and Oriental Medicine
www.ccaom.org

International Qigong Alliance
www.qigong-alliance.org

Jin Shin Do Foundation for
Bodymind Acupressure
http://jinshindo.org

National Qigong Association
www.nqa.org

Qigong Association of America
www.qi.org

Qigong Institute
www.qigonginstitute.org

Society for Acupuncture Research
www.acupunctureresearch.org

BIOFEEDBACK

Association for Applied
Psychophysiology and Biofeedback
www.aapb.org

Biofeedback Foundation of Europe
www.bfe.org

BODYMIND CONNECTEDNESS

Academy of Psychosomatic Medicine
www.apm.org

American Institute of Stress
www.stress.org

American Psychosomatic Society
www.psychosomatic.org

Association for Research in Nervous
and Mental Disease
www.arnmd.org

Benson-Henry Institute for Mind
Body Medicine
www.massgeneral.org/bhi

Canadian Institute of Stress
www.stresscanada.org

Center for Mind-Body Research
(Johns Hopkins University)
www.jhsph.edu/mindbodyresearch

Center for Mindfulness in Medicine,
Health Care, and Society (University
of Massachusetts Medical School)
www.umassmed.edu/Content
.aspx?id=41252

Cousins Center for
Psychoneuroimmunology (University
of California—Los Angeles)
www.semel.ucla.edu/cousins

Institute of HeartMath
www.heartmath.org

International College of
Psychosomatic Medicine
www.icpm.org

Psychoneuroimmunology Research
Society
www.pnirs.org

Royal College of Medicine—
Hypnosis and Psychosomatic
Medicine Section
www.rsm.ac.uk/academ/sech_p.php

Society for Psychophysiological
Research
http://sprweb.org

CHRONIC FATIGUE SYNDROME

CFIDS (Chronic Fatigue and
Immune Dysfunction) Association of
America
www.cfids.org

Chronic Syndrome Support Assoc.
www.cssa-inc.org

International Assoc. for CFS/ME
www.iacfsme.org

National CFIDS (Chronic Fatigue and
Immune Dysfunction) Foundation
www.ncf-net.org

National Chronic Fatigue Syndrome
and Fibromyalgia Association
www.ncfsfa.org

CHRONIC PAIN/PHANTOM PAIN

American Academy of Pain
Management
www.aapainmanage.org

American Academy of Pain Medicine
www.painmed.org

American Chronic Pain Association
www.theacpa.org

American Pain Foundation
www.painfoundation.org

American Pain Society
www.ampainsoc.org

Canadian Pain Society
www.canadianpainsociety.ca

Chronic Pain Association of Canada
www.chronicpaincanada.com

Chronic Pain Research Alliance
http://overlappingconditions.org

International Association for the
Study of Pain
www.iasp-pain.org

Jaw Joints and Allied Musculo-Skeletal Disorders Foundation
www.tmjoints.org

National Chronic Pain Outreach Association
www.chronicpain.org

Phantom Pain Syndrome Association
http://phantompainsyndrome.org

TMJ (Temperomandibular Joint) Association
www.tmj.org

UCLA Center for Neurovisceral Sciences and Women's Health
www.cns.med.ucla.edu/index-women-shealth.htm

FIBROMYALGIA/RHEUMATOID ARTHRITIS

American College of Rheumatology
www.rheumatology.org

American Fibromyalgia Syndrome Association
www.afsafund.org

Arthritis National Research Foundation
www.curearthritis.org

British Society for Rheumatology
www.rheumatology.org.uk

Chronic Syndrome Support Association
www.cssa-inc.org

Fibromyalgia Coalition International
http://fibrocoalition.org

Fibromyalgia Network
www.fmnetnews.com

The FMS Community
www.fmscommunity.org

International Myopain Society
www.myopain.org

National Chronic Fatigue Syndrome and Fibromyalgia Association
www.ncfsfa.org

National Fibromyalgia Association
www.fmaware.org

National Fibromyalgia Partnership
www.fmpartnership.org

National Fibromyalgia Research Association
www.nfra.net

National Rheumatoid Arthritis Society (UK)
www.nras.org.uk

Overlapping Conditions Alliance
http://overlappingconditions.org

UK Fibromyalgia
www.ukfibromyalgia.com

GUIDED IMAGERY

Academy for Guided Imagery
www.acadgi.com

Imagery International
http://imageryinternational.org

HIGHLY SENSITIVE (VERY THIN BOUNDARY) PEOPLE

The Highly Sensitive Person
www.hsperson.com

Highly Sensitive Person Connections
www.hspconnections.com

HYPERTENSION

American Heart Association—High Blood Pressure
www.heart.org

American Society of Hypertension
www.ash-us.org

British Hypertension Society
www.bhsoc.org

European Society of Hypertension
www.eshonline.org

Hypertension Canada
www.hypertension.ca

Hypertension Education Foundation
www.hypertensionfoundation.org

International Pediatric Hypertension Association
www.pediatrichypertension.org

International Society of Hypertension
www.ish-world.com

International Society on Hypertension in Blacks
www.ishib.org

National Alliance to Reach Blood Pressure Goals
www.fromatoa.org

National Hypertension Association
www.nathypertension.org

World Hypertension League
www.worldhypertensionleague.org

HYPNOTHERAPY

American Association of Professional Hypnotherapists
www.aaph.org

American Hypnosis Association
www.hypnosis.edu

American Psychotherapy and Medical Hypnosis Association
http://apmha.com

American Society of Clinical Hypnosis
www.asch.net

Association of Registered Clinical Hypnotherapists (CAN)
www.archcanada.ca

British Society of Clinical and Academic Hypnosis
www.bscah.com

British Society of Clinical Hypnosis
www.bsch.org.uk

Canadian Federation of Clinical Hypnosis
http://clinicalhypnosis.ca

European Society of Hypnosis
http://esh-hypnosis.eu

Hypnosis and Hypnotherapy (UK)
www.hypnosis.me.uk

Hypnotherapy Association (UK)
www.thehypnotherapyassociation.co.uk

Hypnotherapy Society (UK)
www.hypnotherapysociety.com

IBSHypnosis.com
www.ibshypnosis.com

International Association of Hypnoanalysts (UK)
www.hypnoanalysis.com

International Medical and Dental Hypnotherapy Association
www.imdha.com

International Society of Hypnosis
www.ish-hypnosis.org

National Council for Hypnotherapy (UK)
www.hypnotherapists.org.uk

Royal College of Medicine— Hypnosis and Psychosomatic Medicine Section
www.rsm.ac.uk/academ/sech_p.php

Society for Clinical and Experimental Hypnosis
www.sceh.us

Society of Psychological Hypnosis (Division 30 of the American Psychological Association)
http://psychologicalhypnosis.com

IMMUNE DISORDERS/ ENVIRONMENTAL HEALTH

American Academy of Environmental Medicine
www.aaemonline.org

American Autoimmune Related Diseases Association
www.aarda.org

American Environmental Health Foundation
www.aehf.com

Canadian Immunodeficiencies Patient Organization
http://cipo.ca/English.html

Immune Deficiency Foundation
www.primaryimmune.org

Immune Tolerance Network
www.immunetolerance.org

International Society of Developmental and Comparative Immunology
www.isdci.org

Primary Immunodeficiency Network (UK)
www.ukpin.org.uk

IRRITABLE BOWEL SYNDROME/ULCER

American College of Gastroenterology
www.acg.gi.org

American Gastroenterological Association
www.gastro.org

American Neurogastroenterology and Motility Society
www.motilitysociety.org

British Society of Gastroenterology
www.bsg.org.uk

Canadian Association of Gastroenterology
www.cag-acg.org

Crohn's and Colitis Foundation of America
www.ccfa.org

Crohn's and Colitis Foundation of Canada
www.ccfc.ca

Digestive Disorders Foundation (UK)
www.digestivedisorders.org.uk

European Pressure Ulcer Advisory Panel
www.epuap.org

The Gut Trust (Formerly IBS Network—UK)
www.ibsnetwork.org.uk

IBSHypnosis.com
www.ibshypnosis.com

IBS Self Help and Support Group
www.ibsgroup.org

International Foundation for Functional Gastrointestinal Disorders
www.iffgd.org

Irritable Bowel Syndrome Association
www.ibsassociation.org

Irritable Bowel Syndrome Self Help and Support Group
www.ibsgroup.org

National Pressure Ulcer Advisory Panel
www.npuap.org

Overlapping Conditions Alliance
http://overlappingconditions.org

UCLA Center for Neurovisceral Sciences and Women's Health
www.cns.med.ucla.edu/index-women-shealth.htm

UNC Center for Functional GI and Motility Disorders (University of North Carolina—Chapel Hill)
www.med.unc.edu/medicine/fgidc

United European Gastroenterology Federation
www.uegf.org

MEDITATION/STRESS REDUCTION/ YOGA

Benson-Henry Institute for Mind Body Medicine
www.massgeneral.org/bhi

British Meditation Society
www.britishmeditationsociety.org

Center for Mindfulness (University of Massachusetts Medical School)
www.umassmed.edu/cfm/stress/index.aspx

International Association of Yoga Therapists
www.iayt.org

Meditation Society of America
www.meditationsociety.com

Mindfulness Based Stress Reduction (directory of programs worldwide)
http://w3.umassmed.edu/MBSR/public/searchmember.aspx

Vipassana Dhura Meditation Society
www.vipassanadhura.com

MIGRAINE

American Headache Society
www.americanheadachesociety.org

Committee for Headache Education
www.achenet.org

Headache Network Canada
www.headachenetwork.ca

MAGNUM, the Migraine Awareness Group
www.migraines.org

Migraine Action (UK)
www.migraine.org.uk

The Migraine Trust (UK)
www.migrainetrust.org

National Headache Foundation
www.headaches.org

World Headache Alliance
www.w-h-a.org

PERSONALITY RESEARCH

Assoc. for Humanistic Psychology
www.ahpweb.org

Association for Humanistic Psychology in Britain
www.ahpb.org.uk

Assoc. for Research in Personality
www.personality-arp.org

European Association of Personality Psychology
www.eapp.org

European Association of Psychological Assessment
www.eapa-homepage.org

International Society for the Study of Individual Differences
www.issid.org

International Society for the Study of Personality Disorders
www.isspd.com

Society for Humanistic Psychology (Division 32 of the American Psychological Association)
www.apa.org/divisions/div32

Society for Personality and Social Psychology
www.spsp.org

Society for Personality Assessment
www.personality.org

UK Association of Humanistic Psychology Practitioners
www.ahpp.org

POST-TRAUMATIC STRESS DISORDER

American Academy of Experts in Traumatic Stress
www.aaets.org

American Trauma Society
www.amtrauma.org

Association of Traumatic Stress Specialists
www.atss.info

European Society for Traumatic Stress Studies
www.estss.org

International Society for Traumatic Stress Studies
www.istss.org

International Trauma Healing Institute
www.traumainstitute.org

National Center for PTSD
www.ncptsd.va.gov

National Neurotrauma Society
www.neurotraumasociety.org

PTSD Alliance
www.ptsdalliance.org

Sidran Institute
www.sidran.org

Somatic Experiencing Trauma Institute
www.traumahealing.com

Traumatic Incident Reduction Association
www.tir.org

Traumatic Stress Group (CAN)
www.ttsg.ca

PSORIASIS/ECZEMA

International Federation of Psoriasis Associations
www.ifpa-pso.org

National Eczema Association
www.nationaleczema.org

National Eczema Society (UK)
www.eczema.org

National Psoriasis Foundation
www.psoriasis.org

Psoriasis Association (UK)
www.psoriasis-association.org.uk

Psoriasis Help Organization (UK)
www.psoriasis-help.org.uk

Psoriasis International Network
http://psoriasis-international.org

Psoriasis Society of Canada
www.psoriasissociety.org

SOMATIC AND ENERGY THERAPIES

American Massage Therapy Assoc.
www.amtamassage.org

American Polarity Therapy Assoc.
www.polaritytherapy.org

American Society for the Alexander Technique
www.alexandertech.org

Associated Bodywork and Massage Professionals
www.abmp.com

Association for the Advancement of Meridian Energy Techniques
www.aamet.org

Association for Comprehensive Energy Psychology
www.energypsych.org

Association for Holotropic Breathwork International
www.grof-holotropic-breathwork.net

Association for Meridian Energy Therapies
http://theamt.com

Association of Holistic Biodynamic Massage Therapists (UK)
www.ahbmt.org

Association of Reflexologists (UK)
www.aor.org.uk

Authentic Movement Institute
www.authenticmovement-usa.com

Biodynamic Craniosacral Therapy Association of North America
www.craniosacraltherapy.org

Body-Mind Centering Association
https://bmcassociation.org

Bodynamic Institute USA
www.bodynamicusa.com

Bowen Therapy/Bowen Technique
www.bowenwork.com

Bowenwork Academy USA
www.bowenworkacademyusa.com

British Reflexology Association
www.britreflex.co.uk

Cambridge Body Psychotherapy Centre (UK)
www.cbpc.org.uk

Canadian Association for Integrative and Energy Therapies
www.caiet.org

Canadian Massage and Acupressure Therapists Association
http://catamassage.org

Canadian Reiki Association
www.reiki.ca

Chiron Association for Body Psychotherapists (UK)
www.body-psychotherapy.org.uk

Craniosacral Therapy Association of the UK
www.craniosacral.co.uk

EFT (Emotional Freedom Technique) Founding Masters
www.eftmastersworldwide.com

EMDR (Eye Movement Desensitization and Reprocessing) Institute
www.emdr.com

EMDR Canada
www.emdrcanada.org

EMDR Europe
http://emdr-europe.org

EMDR International Association
www.emdria.org

Energy Kinesiology Association
www.energyk.org

Energy Therapy Net
www.meridiantherapy.org

European Association for Body Psychotherapy
www.eabp.org

European Rolfing Association
www.rolfing.org

Federation of Holistic Therapists (UK)
www.fht.org.uk

Feldenkrais Educational Foundation of North America
www.feldenkrais.com

Feldenkrais Guild of North America
www.feldenkrais.com

Feldenkrais Guild (UK)
www.feldenkrais.co.uk

Feldenkrais Movement Institute
www.feldenkraisinstitute.org

Focusing Institute
www.focusing.org

General Council for Massage Therapies (UK)
www.gcmt.org.uk

Guild for Structural Integration
www.rolfguild.org

Hakomi Institute
www.hakomiinstitute.com

Healing Touch International
www.healingtouch.net

Healing Touch Professional Assoc.
www.htprofessionalassociation.com

Healing Touch Program
www.healingtouchprogram.com

Hellerwork Structural Integration
www.hellerwork.com

International Association of Reiki Professionals
www.iarp.org

International Breathwork Foundation
www.ibfnetwork.com

International Breathwork Training Alliance
http://breathworkalliance.com

International Council of Reflexologists
www.icr-reflexology.org

International Federation of Reflexologists
www.intfedreflexologists.org

International Institute for Bioenergetic Analysis
www.bioenergetic-therapy.com

International Somatic Movement Education and Therapy Association
www.ismeta.org

Massage Therapy Canada
www.massage.ca

Massage Therapy UK
http://massagetherapy.co.uk

National Association of Massage and Manipulative Therapists (UK)
www.nammt.co.uk

National Association of Massage Therapists
http://namtonline.com

National Association of Myofascial Trigger Point Therapists
www.myofascialtherapy.org

Nurse Healers Professional Associates International
www.therapeutic-touch.org

Reflexology Association of America
www.reflexology-usa.org

Reflexology Association of Canada
www.reflexolog.org

Reiki Alliance
www.reikialliance.com

Reiki Association (UK)
www.reikiassociation.org.uk

Rosen Institute
www.rosenmethod.org

Rosen Method Professional
Association
http://rmpa.net

Rubenfeld Synergy Method
www.rubenfeldsynergy.com

Sensorimotor Psychotherapy
Institute
www.sensorimotorpsychotherapy.org

Shiatsu Society (UK)
www.shiatsusociety.org

Society of Teachers of the Alexander
Technique (UK)
www.stat.org.uk

Somatic Experiencing Trauma
Institute
www.traumahealing.com

Touch Research Institute
www6.miami.edu/touch-research

TragerCanada
www.trager/ca

Trager International
www.trager.com

Trager UK
www.trager.co.uk

UK Polarity Therapy Association
www.polarity.tk

United States Association for Body
Psychotherapy
www.usabp.org

United States Trager Association
www.trager-us.org

Upledger Institute
www.upledger.com

World Reiki Association
www.worldreikiassociation.org

Zero Balancing Association UK
www.zerobalancinguk.org

Zero Balancing Health Association
www.zerobalancing.com

WOMEN'S HEALTH

Center for Women's Health
www.centerforwomenshealth.com

Centres of Excellence for Women's
Health (CAN)
www.cewh-cesf.ca/en/index.shtml

National Assoc. for Women's Health
http://nawh.org

National Women's Health Network
www.nwhn.org

National Women's Health Resource
Center
www.healthywomen.org

Office of Research on Women's Health
(National Institutes of Health)
http://orwh.od.nih.gov

Office on Women's Health (U.S.
Department of Health and Human
Services)
www.womenshealth.gov

Organization for the Study of Sex
Differences
www.ossdweb.org

Society for Women's Health Research
www.womenshealthresearch.org

UCLA Center for Neurovisceral
Sciences and Women's Health
www.cns.med.ucla.edu/index-
womenshealth.htm

Women's Health America
www.womenshealth.com

Women's Health Matters (CAN)
www.womenshealthmatters.ca

NOTES

FOREWORD

1. United States Department of Health and Human Services, National Health Statistics Reports, no. 18 (July 30, 2009).

INTRODUCTION

1. Elias and Ketcham, *The Five Elements of Self-Healing,* 282.
2. Morris, *American Heritage Dictionary of the English Language,* 1324.
3. Rosch, "Some Psychological Perspectives on Traits, Temperament and Personality," 8.
4. Nahin et al., *Costs of Complementary and Alternative Medicine,* 1.
5. "Doctors, Nurses Often Use Holistic Medicine for Themselves."
6. Topf with Bennett, *You Are Not Your Illness,* 22.
7. Chapman, "Pain, Suffering, and the Self."
8. Elias and Ketcham, *The Five Elements of Self-Healing,* 282–83.
9. Jung, *An Answer to Job,* quoted in Juhan, *Job's Body,* 19.

CHAPTER 1. YOU ARE YOUR BODYMIND

1. Morris, *American Heritage Dictionary of the English Language,* 978.
2. "'Life Force' Linked to Body's Ability to Withstand Stress."
3. Cloninger, *Feeling Good: The Science of Well-Being.*
4. Kundera, *Immortality,* 204.
5. Dychtwald, *Bodymind.*
6. Gershon, *The Second Brain,* xiii.
7. Martin, *The Healing Mind,* 68–69.
8. Pert, *Molecules of Emotion,* 143, 185.
9. Gershon, *The Second Brain,* xiii.

10. Ibid.

11. Pearce, *Evolution's End,* 104.

12. "Science of the Heart."

13. Oschman, *Energy Medicine,* 29; Pearsall, *The Heart's Code,* 55, 65.

14. Watkins, "The Electrical Heart," 305–18.

15. Damasio, *Descartes' Error,* 159.

16. Humphrey, *A History of the Mind,* 115.

17. Bachner-Melman et al., "*AVPR1a* and *SLC64A* Gene Polymorphisms Are Associated with Creative Dance Performance."

18. Micozzi, *Fundamentals of Complementary and Alternative Medicine,* 4th ed.

CHAPTER 2. OUR BOUNDARIES, OUR SELVES

1. Appel, "Notes on the Psychosomatic Element of Migraine," 209–18.

2. Ibid., 209–18.

3. Greenspan, *Healing through the Dark Emotions,* 219, 231.

4. Sewall, "The Skill of Ecological Perception," 214.

5. Hillman, "A Psyche the Size of the Earth," xvii.

6. Humphrey, *A History of the Mind,* 42–45.

7. Hartmann, *Boundaries in the Mind,* 4–7.

8. Hartmann, Harrison, and Zborowski, "Boundaries in the Mind," 347–68.

9. Aron, *The Highly Sensitive Person.*

10. Kagan and Snidman, *The Long Shadow of Temperament.*

11. Kurcinka, *Raising Your Spirited Child.*

12. Wilson and Barber, "The Fantasy-Prone Personality," 340–87.

13. Heller, *Too Loud, Too Bright, Too Fast, Too Tight.*

14. Lynch, *The Language of the Heart;* Maté, *When the Body Says No.*

15. Aron, *The Highly Sensitive Person,* 7.

16. Lynch, *The Language of the Heart,* 209–13, 220–22.

17. Twain, *Following the Equator.*

18. Sacks, quoted in Appel, "Notes on the Psychosomatic Element of Migraine," 209–18.

19. Appel, "Notes on the Psychosomatic Element of Migraine," 209–18.

20. Hartmann, *Boundaries in the Mind,* 236.

21. Appel, "Notes on the Psychosomatic Element of Migraine," 209–18.

22. Schulz, *Awakening Intuition,* 102.

23. Broom, *Somatic Illness and the Patient's Other Story,* 172.

24. Montagu, *Touching,* 2nd ed., 4.

25. Ibid., 2.

26. Montagu, *Touching,* 3rd ed., 272.

CHAPTER 3. PERSONALITY DIFFERENCES:
A KEY TO DECODING CHRONIC ILLNESS

1. Velle, "Sex Differences in Sensory Functions," 490–522; Schirber, "Women Suffer More Than Men."

2. "Gender Differences in Response to Pain."

3. Lovejoy, "Models of Human Evolution," 304–6.

4. "Brain Imaging Shows How Men and Women Cope Differently under Stress."

5. Lloyd, "Emotional Wiring Different in Men and Women."

6. Durden-Smith and DeSimone, *Sex and the Brain,* 76.

7. Ibid., 77–81; Cocke, "Men and Women Remember Things in Different Ways," 7.

8. Carey, "Men and Women Really Do Think Differently."

9. Cahill, "His Brain, Her Brain," 40–47.

10. "Sex Differences in the Brain's Serotonin System"; "Women More Depressed and Men More Impulsive with Reduced Serotonin Functioning"; "One Gene Variant Puts Stressed Women at Risk for Depression; Has Opposite Effect in Men."

11. McManamy, "Depression in Women."

12. Begley, "The Depressing News about Antidepressants," 40.

13. Paddock, "Retrovirus Linked to Chronic Fatigue Syndrome."

14. "New Virus Is Not Linked to Chronic Fatigue Syndrome"; "Further Doubt Cast on Virus Link to Chronic Fatigue"; "Chronic Fatigue Syndrome Not Related to XMRV Retrovirus, Comprehensive Study Finds."

15. "*Helicobacter pylori* and Peptic Ulcer Disease"; Currey, "Research in the News: Ulcers"; O'Connor, *Undoing Perpetual Stress,* 350.

16. Yunus, "Are Fibromyalgia and Other Chronic Conditions Associated?"

17. Solomon, "Psychoneuroimmunology and Chronic Fatigue Syndrome," 7.

18. Martin, *The Healing Mind,* 134–35.

19. Montagu, *Touching,* 3rd ed., 272.

20. Gilbert, "Breaking the Paradigm."

CHAPTER 4. BOUNDARY SIMILARITIES AND DIFFERENCES:
CHRONIC FATIGUE, PTSD, IRRITABLE BOWEL, AND FIBROMYALIGIA

1. Reeves, *Women's Intuition,* xi.

2. Griffin, *What Her Body Thought.*

3. Ibid., 21–22.

4. Ibid., 43.

5. Ibid., 37.

6. Ibid., 37–38, 44.

7. Ibid., 29, 41, 48, 73.

8. Hartmann, Harrison, and Zborowski, "Boundaries in the Mind, " 347–68.

9. Berne, *Chronic Fatigue Syndrome, Fibromyalgia, and Other Invisible Illnesses,* 118.

10. Maté, *When the Body Says No.*

11. "Chronic Fatigue Patients Show Lower Response to Placebos."

12. Pearson, "Chronic Fatigue Has Genetic Roots"; Gardner, "Genetics May Drive Chronic Fatigue Syndrome"; Maugh, "Chronic Fatigue Is in the Genes," A1; See, "New Evidence That Genetics Are Responsible for Chronic Fatigue Syndrome."

13. Nathanielsz, *Life in the Womb,* 126–7.

14. Ibid., 130.

15. DeNoon, "Childhood Trauma Raises CFS Risk"; "Childhood Trauma and Chronic Fatigue Syndrome Risk Biologically Linked"; Boyles, "CFC Linked to Childhood Trauma."

16. DeNoon, "Childhood Trauma Raises CFS Risk."

17. "New Hypothesis Proposed for Cause of Chronic Fatigue Syndrome."

18. "Post Traumatic Stress Disorder Fact Sheet."

19. Yehuda, "Psychoneuroendocrinology of Post-Traumatic Stress Disorder," 359–79; Heim et al., "Pituitary-Adrenal and Autonomic Responses to Stress in Women After Sexual and Physical Abuse in Childhood," 592–97; Pfeffer et al., "Salivary Cortisol and Psychopathology in Children Bereaved by the September 11, 2001 Terror Attacks," 957–65; Van Den Eede et al., "Hypothalamic-Pituitary-Adrenal Axis Function in Chronic Fatigue Syndrome," 112–20; Silverman et al., "Neuroendocrine and Immune Contributors to Fatigue," 338–46; Demitrack and Crofford, "Evidence for and Pathophysiological Implications of Hypothalamic-Pituitary-Adrenal Axis Dysregulation in Fibromyalgia and Chronic Fatigue Syndrome," 684–97.

20. Sharpe et al., "Increased Brain Serotonin Function in Men with Chronic Fatigue Syndrome," 164–65; Parker, Wessely, and Cleare, "The Neuroendocrinology of Chronic Fatigue Syndrome and Fibromyalgia," 1331–45; Arora et al., "Paroxetine Binding in the Blood Platelets of Post-Traumatic Stress Disorder Patients," 919–28; Connor and Butterfield, "Post Traumatic Stress Disorder," 247–62.

21. Shin et al., "Regional Cerebral Blood Flow During Script-Driven Imagery

in Childhood Sexual Abuse-Related PTSD," 575–84; Medow, "Going with the Flow—Blood Flow, That Is;" Vernon, "Association-Funded Researchers Making Headway."

22. Kline and Rausch, "Olfactory Precipitants of Flashback in Posttraumatic Stress Disorder," 383–84.
23. "Brain Response Differences in the Way Women with IBS Anticipate and React to Pain."
24. "Abuse History Affects Pain Regulation in Women with Irritable Bowel Syndrome."
25. Brown, "A Brain in the Head, and One in the Gut."
26. "Mayo Clinic Researchers Find Link between Irritable Bowel Syndrome (IBS), Alcoholism and Mental Illness"; "Irritable Bowel Syndrome's Possible Genetic Link Studied."
27. "Overly Anxious and Driven People Prone to Irritable Bowel Syndrome."
28. "Allergic Disease Linked to Irritable Bowel Syndrome."
29. Cole et al., "Migraine, Fibromyalgia, and Depression among People with IBS."
30. Hadhazy, "Think Twice: How the Gut's 'Second Brain' Influences Mood and Well Being."
31. Sharpe et al., "Increased Brain Serotonin Function in Men with Chronic Fatigue Syndrome," 164–65; Parker, Wessely, and Cleare, "The Neuroendocrinology of Chronic Fatigue Syndrome and Fibromyalgia," 1331–45; "Irritable Bowel Syndrome," National Digestive Diseases Information Clearinghouse; F. Wolfe et al., "Serotonin Levels, Pain Threshold, and Fibromyalgia Symptoms in the General Population," 555–59; Juhl, "Fibromyalgia and the Serotonin Pathway," 367–75; Nicolodi and Sicuteri, "Fibromyalgia and Migraine, Two Faces of the Same Mechanism," 373–79.
32. "Fibromyalgia Syndrome," *Health and Stress,* 2.
33. Yunus, "Are Fibromyalgia and Other Chronic Conditions Associated?"
34. Chaitow, "Chronic Fatigue/Fibromyalgia."
35. Berne, *Chronic Fatigue Syndrome, Fibromyalgia, and Other Invisible Illnesses,* 92; Sperber et al., "Fibromyalgia in the Irritable Bowel Syndrome," 3541–46.
36. "Headaches and Fibromyalgia"; "Migraine and Fibromyalgia May Affect Nearly One-Quarter of Female Migraineurs."
37. Juhl, "Fibromyalgia and the Serotonin Pathway," 367–75; Russell et al., "Cerebrospinal Fluid Biogenic Amine Metabolites in Fibromyalgia/Fibrositis Syndrome and Rheumatoid Arthritis," 550–56; "Irritable Bowel Syndrome,"

National Digestive Diseases Information Clearinghouse; Wolfe et al., "Serotonin Levels, Pain Threshold, and Fibromyalgia Symptoms in the General Population," 555–59.

38. Boyles, "Posttraumatic Stress, Fibromyalgia Linked;" Amir et al., "Posttraumatic Stress Disorder, Tenderness and Fibromyalgia," 607–13.

39. Weissbecker et al., "Childhood Trauma and Dirurnal Cortisol Disruption in Fibromyalgia Syndrome," 312–24; Van Houdenhove et al., "Victimization in Chronic Fatigue Syndrome and Fibromyalgia in Tertiary Care," 21–28.

40. Scaer, "Observations on Traumatic Stress."

CHAPTER 5. FEELINGS ON HOLD:
DEPRESSION, HYPERTENSION, MIGRAINE, AND PHANTOM PAIN

1. Lynch, *The Language of the Heart,* 14–20.

2. Ibid., 23–28.

3. Ibid., 210–11.

4. Ibid., 210–13.

5. Meuret et al., "Do Unexpected Panic Attacks Occur Spontaneously?"

6. Lynch, The Language of the Heart, 210–16.

7. Ibid., 209.

8. Ford, *Compassionate Touch,* 214.

9. Broom, *Meaning*-Full *Disease,* 2–4.

10. Ibid., 7.

11. Appel, "Notes on the Psychosomatic Element of Migraine," 209–18.

12. Lance, *Migraines and Other Headaches,* 89.

13. "Migraine Headache Overview, Types of Migraine."

14. "Adverse Childhood Experiences Linked to Frequent Headache in Adults"; "Abuse in Childhood Linked to Migraine and Other Pain Disorders;" Tietjen et al., "Childhood Maltreatment and Migraine (Part II)," 32–41.

15. "Migraine Headaches"; "Understanding Migraines."

16. Lynch, *The Language of the Heart,* 222.

17. Medow, "Going with the Flow"; Vernon, "Association-Funded Researchers Making Headway."

18. Streeten and Bell, "Circulating Blood Volume in Chronic Fatigue Syndrome," 3–11.

19. Kansky, "New Treatment for NMH."

20. Bell, "The Lyndonville Journal: Evaluating Blood Volume Studies."

21. Eden with Feinstein, *Energy Medicine,* 18.

22. Broom, *Meaning*-Full *Disease*, 114–15.

23. "Asthma Linked to Post-Traumatic Stress Disorder."

24. Jawer with Micozzi, *The Spiritual Anatomy of Emotion*, 227–28, 348–49.

25. Melzack, "Phantom Limbs," 120–26.

26. Leskowitz, "Phantom Pain," 125–52.

27. Ibid.

28. O'Connor, *Undoing Perpetual Stress*, 350.

29. Melzack, "Phantom Limbs," 84–91.

30. Lynch, *The Language of the Heart*, 226–27.

31. Sifneos, "The Prevalence of 'Alexithymic' Characteristics," 255–62.

32. Muller, "When a Patient Has No Story to Tell," 71–72.

33. MacClaren, "Emotional Disorder and the Mind-Body Problem," 139–55.

34. Hartmann, *Dreams and Nightmares*, 287–88.

35. Sifneos, "The Prevalence of 'Alexithymic' Characteristics," 255–62.

36. Hartmann, *Dreams and Nightmares*, 287–88; MacClaren, "Emotional Disorder and the Mind-Body Problem," 139–55.

37. Muller, "When a Patient Has No Story to Tell," 71–72.

38. McDougall, *Theaters of the Mind*, 165.

39. Ibid., 169, 175–76.

40. MacClaren, "Emotional Disorder and the Mind-Body Problem," 139–55; Todarello et al., "Alexithymia in Essential Hypertensive and Psychiatric Outpatients," 987–94; Jula, Salminen, and Saarijärvi, "Alexithymia: A Facet of Essential Hypertension," 1057–61; Serrano et al., "Alexithymia: A Relevant Psychological Variable in Near-Fatal Asthma," 296–302; Kosturek et al., "Alexithymia and Somatic Amplification in Chronic Pain," 399–404; Van de Putte et al., "Alexithymia in Adolescents with Chronic Fatigue Syndrome," 377–80; Jones et al., "Alexithymia and Somatosensory Amplification in Functional Dyspepsia," 508–16.

41. Hill, Berthoz, and Frith, "Brief Report: Cognitive Processing of Own Emotions," 229–35; Fitzgerald and Bellgrove, "The Overlap between Alexithymia and Asperger's Syndrome," 573–76.

42. Robotham, "Brain Link to Fatigue Syndrome."

43. "Is the Inability to Express Emotions Hereditary?"

44. Koponen et al., "Alexithymia after Traumatic Brain Injury," 807–12.

45. Lynch, *The Language of the Heart*, 221.

46. MacClaren, "Emotional Disorder and the Mind-Body Problem," 139–55; McDougall, *Theaters of the Body*, 94.

47. Lynch, *The Language of the Heart*, 274.

48. "National Survey Sharpens Picture of Major Depression among U.S. Adults."

49. Axe et al., "Major Depressive Disorder in Chronic Fatigue Syndrome," 7–23; Wallace and Wallace, *All about Fibromyalgia,* 188.

50. O'Connor, *Undoing Perpetual Stress.*

51. McManamy, "FDA Antidepressant Suicide Warning."

52. Frattaroli, *Healing the Soul in the Age of the Brain.*

CHAPTER 6. FINDING YOUR BOUNDARY TYPE

1. Ernest Hartmann, correspondence with author, November 13, 2003.

2. Hartmann, *Dreams and Nightmares,* 228.

3. Ibid., 229.

4. Hartmann, Harrison, and Zborowski, "Boundaries in the Mind, "347–68; Karen Wyman, correspondence with Michael Jawer, May 4, 2010.

5. Hartmann, Harrison, and Zborowski, "Boundaries in the Mind," 347–68.

6. Ibid.

7. Ibid.

8. McCrae and Costa, "Conceptions and Correlates of Openness to Experience," 825–47.

9. Hartmann, Harrison, and Zborowski, "Boundaries in the Mind," 347–68.

9. Vance, "Seeking to Illuminate the Mysterious Placebo Effect."

CHAPTER 7. FINDING YOUR REMEDY

1. "Allergy Facts and Figures."

2. "Diseases 101."

3. Asthma and Allergy Foundation of America, "Allergy Facts and Figures."

4. Hajjar, Kotchen, and Kotchen, "Hypertension," 465–90; Kaplan, "The Prevalence and Control of Hypertension."

5. "American Migraine Prevalence and Prevention;" Center for the Advancement of Health, *Facts of Life.*

6. Stewart et al., "Prevalence of Migraine Headache in the United States," 64–69; Tepper, "Migraine Prevalence and Disease Burden."

7. "Prevalence."

8. "Diagnosis: Do I Have CFS?"

9. Boivin, "Socioeconomic Impact of Irritable Bowel Syndrome in Canada," 8B–11B.

10. Kessler et al., "Posttraumatic Stress Disorder in the National Comorbidity Survey," 1048–60.

11. "National Survey Sharpens Picture of Major Depression among U.S. Adults."

12. Nahin et al., Costs of Complementary and Alternative Medicine, 1.

13. Micozzi, Fundamentals of Complementary and Alternative Medicine, 4th ed.

14. Whalley, "Measurement of Hypnosis and Hypnotisability."

15. Hartmann, Harrison, and Zborowski, "Boundaries in the Mind," 347–68.

16. Jawer with Micozzi, The Spiritual Anatomy of Emotion, 307, 335–36.

17. Cocke, "Men and Women Remember Things in Different Ways," 7.

18. Hartmann, "Boundaries in the Mind," grant proposal.

19. Pert, quoted in Oschman, Energy Medicine, ix.

20. Cardini and Weixin, "Moxibustion for Correction of Breech Presentation," 1580–84; Neri et al., "Acupuncture Plus Moxibustion to Resolve Breech Presentation," 247–52; Vas et al., "Correction of Nonvertex Presentation with Moxibustion," 241–59.

21. McCown and Micozzi, Walking into Now.

22. Toffler, Future Shock.

23. Morris, The Human Zoo.

24. Selye, The Stress of Life.

25. Benson, The Relaxation Response.

CHAPTER 8. PUSHING BOUNDARIES:
TREATMENTS BEYOND THE SUPER SEVEN

1. Morris, American Heritage Dictionary of the English Language, 607, 1520.

2. Kaptchuk, The Web That Has No Weaver, 3–4, 34, 51.

3. Ibid., x–xi, 2–3, 51–52.

4. Kidson, Is Acupuncture Right for You?, 5, 31.

5. Gao, Chinese Medicine, 125.

6. Micozzi, Fundamentals of Complementary and Alternative Medicine, 4th ed., 14.

7. Kidson, Is Acupuncture Right for You?, 32–33, 75.

8. Ibid., 3, 82.

9. Ibid., 40–41.

10. Elias and Ketcham, The Five Elements of Self-Healing, 277–78; Kaptchuk, The Web That Has No Weaver, 42; Co and Roberts with Merryman, Your Hands Can Heal You, 66–67.

11. Kidson, *Is Acupuncture Right for You?* 22, 28, 30–31.

12. Ibid., 166.

13. Servan-Schreiber, *The Instinct to Heal,* 120–21.

14. Diamond, *Life Energy,* 5; Co and Roberts with Merryman, *Your Hands Can Heal You,* 79.

15. Mann, *Acupuncture,* 54–55.

16. Ives and Jonas, "Energy and Medicine," 161–74.

17. Montagu, *Touching,* 2nd ed., 1–2.

18. Field, *Touch,* 98–99.

19. Hover-Kramer, *Creative Energies,* 77–78; Krieger, *Therapeutic Touch as Transpersonal Healing,* 69; Claire, *Bodywork,* 136; Oz with Arias and Oz, *Healing from the Heart,* 119, 126; Rubenfeld, *The Listening Hand,* 18.

20. Claire, *Bodywork,* viii.

21. Ibid., viii, 139, 157; Oz with Arias and Oz, *Healing from the Heart,* 123.

22. Krieger, *Therapeutic Touch as Transpersonal Healing,* 4–5; Bruce, *Miracle Touch,* 21; Field, *Touch,* 97.

23. Kidson, *Is Acupuncture Right for You?,* 5–7.

24. Green et al., "Anomalous Electrostatic Phenomena in Exceptional Subjects," 69–94.

25. Oz with Arias and Oz, *Healing from the Heart,* 121–32.

26. Jawer with Micozzi, *The Spiritual Anatomy of Emotion.*

27. Rubenfeld, *The Listening Hand,* 5.

28. Ibid., 23.

29. Pennebaker, *Opening Up,* 2, 9.

30. Sharples, "Wish Fulfillment?"

31. Claire, *Bodywork,* 110, 128–29, 163.

32. Johnson, "The Primacy of Experiential Practices in Body-Psychotherapy."

33. Nathanielsz, *Life in the Womb;* Paul, *Origins.*

34. Broom, *Meaning-Full Disease,* 75.

35. Claire, *Bodywork,* 60, 102.

36. Carroll, "Why Psychosomatization Is Complex"; Carroll, "Introduction and Background."

37. "The Seven Developmental Stages."

38. Broom, *Meaning-Full Disease,* 168.

39. "The Seven Developmental Stages"; Ford, *Compassionate Touch,* 77–81.

40. Bernhardt and Isaacs, "The Bodymap."

41. Rubenfeld, *The Listening Hand,* 69.

42. Rothschild, *The Body Remembers,* 24.

43. Swaminathan, "A Gene to Better Remember Traumatic Events."
44. Rajamannar Ramasubbu, "The Amnesia Gene."
45. Field, *Touch*, 72–73.
46. Fitch and Dryden, "Recovering Body and Soul from Post-Traumatic Stress Disorder," 41–62.
47. Hollifield et al., "Acupuncture for Posttraumatic Stress Disorder," 504–13; Ford, *Compassionate Touch*, 19–25; Brooke, "The Logic of Bodywork for Dissociation and Traumatic Stress"; Juhan, *Job's Body*, 414–17.
48. Leskowitz, "Energy Medicine Perspectives on Phantom Pain," 59–63.
49. Juhan, *Job's Body*, 5 (emphasis original).
50. Duff, *The Alchemy of Illness*, 33.
51. Ibid., 9.
52. Ibid., 81.
53. Ibid., 65.
54. Elias and Ketcham, *The Five Elements of Self-Healing*, 282.

APPENDIX B. SELECTED STUDIES SUPPORTING THE EFFECTIVENESS OF CAM TREATMENTS FOR THE DOZEN DISCOMFORTS

1. Antonius Schneider, correspondence with author, April 26, 2010; Schneider et al., "Perception of Bodily Sensation as a Predictor of Treatment Response to Acupuncture," 119–25.
2. Mueller et al., "Treatment of Fibromyalgia Incorporating EEG-Driven Stimulation," 933.
3. Norton et al., "Randomized Controlled Trial of Biofeedback for Fecal Incontinence," 1320.
4. Greco, Rudy, and Manzi, "Effects of a Stress-Reduction Program on Psychological Function, Pain, and Physical Function of Systemic Lupus Erythematosus Patients," 625.
5. Lehrer et al., "Biofeedback Treatment in Asthma," 352.
6. Mason and Black, "Allergic Skin Responses Abolished Under Treatment of Asthma and Hay Fever by Hypnosis," 877.
7. Micozzi, *Fundamentals of Complementary and Alternative Medicine*, 4th ed.
8. Ibid.
9. Gordon, "The Fresh Face of Hypnosis: An Old Practice Finds New Uses."
10. Gonsalkorale, Houghton, and Whorwell, "Hypnotherapy in Irritable Bowel Syndrome," 954.

11. Ibid.

12. Mahoney, "Irritable Bowel Syndrome and Hypnotherapy;" Roth, "Irritable Bowel Syndrome and Hypnosis;" Palsson, "Overview of Published Research To Date on Hypnosis for IBS;" Whorwell, "Hypnotherapy for Functional Gastrointestinal Disorders;" "Hypnotherapy Works for Bowel Pain"; "Hypnotherapy 'Can Help' Irritable Bowel Syndrome."

13. Olness and Gardner, *Hypnosis and Hypnotherapy with Children.*

14. Ibid.

15. Barber, *Hypnosis: A Scientific Approach.*

16. Green and Green, *Beyond Biofeedback.*

17. Luria, *The Mind of a Mnemonist.*

18. Jordan and Lenington, "Psychological Correlates of Eidetic Imagery and Induced Anxiety," 31.

19. Barber, "Changing 'Unchangeable' Bodily Processes by Hypnotic Suggestions," 7; White, "Salivation: the Significance of Imagery in its Voluntary Control," 196.

20. Micozzi, *Fundamentals of Complementary and Alternative Medicine*, 4th ed.

21. Miller, "Nurses at Community Hospital Welcome Guided Imagery," 225.

22. Lewandowski, "Patterning of Pain and Power with Guided Imagery, 233.

23. Benson, Kotch, and Crassweller, "Relaxation Response: Bridge between Psychiatry and Medicine," 929.

24. Cooper and Aygen, "Effects of Meditation on Blood Cholesterol and Blood Pressure," 1.

25. Brooks and Scarano, "Transcendental Meditation in the Treatment of Post-Vietnam Adjustment," 212.

26. Kabat-Zinn et al., "Four-Year Follow-Up of a Meditation-Based Program for the Self-Regulation of Chronic Pain," 163.

27. Schneider et al., "A Randomized Controlled Trial of Stress Reduction for Hypertension in Older African Americans," 820.

28. Kabat-Zinn, "Meditation" in *Healing and the Mind;* Kabat-Zinn, "Mindfulness Meditation" in *Mind-Body Medicine;* McCown, Reibel, and Micozzi, *Teaching Mindfulness.*

29. Kaplan et al., "The Impact of a Meditation-Based Stress Reduction Program on Fibromyalgia," 284.

30. Leskowitz, "Energy Medicine Perspectives on Phantom-Limb Pain," 59–63.

31. Micozzi, *Fundamentals of Complementary and Alternative Medicine,* 4th ed.

32. Ibid.

33. Ibid.

BIBLIOGRAPHY

"Abuse in Childhood Linked to Migraine and Other Pain Disorders." ScienceDaily .org, January 5, 2010. www.sciencedaily.com/releases/2010/01/100106003608. htm. Accessed June 29, 2011.

"Abuse History Affects Pain Regulation in Women with Irritable Bowel Syndrome." ScienceDaily.org, February 3, 2008. www.sciencedaily.com/ releases/2008/02/080201085752.htm. Accessed June 29, 2011.

"Adverse Childhood Experiences Linked to Frequent Headache in Adults." ScienceDaily.com. www.sciencedaily.com/releases/2010/06/100623085518 .htm. Accessed June 29, 2011.

"Allergic Disease Linked to Irritable Bowel Syndrome." ScienceDaily.org, January 31, 2008. www.sciencedaily.com/releases/2008/01/080130170325.htm. Accessed June 29, 2011.

"Allergy Facts and Figures." Asthma and Allergy Foundation of America.org. www .aafa.org/display.cfm?id=9&sub=30. Accessed June 29, 2011.

"American Migraine Prevalence and Prevention (AMPP) Study Fact Sheet." National Headache Foundation. www.headaches.org/press/NHF_Press_Kits/ Press_Kits_-_AMPPS_Fact_Sheet. Accessed June 29, 2011.

Amir, M., et al. "Posttraumatic Stress Disorder, Tenderness and Fibromyalgia." *Journal of Psychosomatic Research* 42, no. 6 (June 1997): 607–13.

Appel, Stephen. "Notes on the Psychosomatic Element of Migraine." *Forum: The Journal of the New Zealand Association of Psychotherapists* 5, no. 3 (1998): 209–18.

Aron, Elaine. *The Highly Sensitive Person: How to Thrive When the World Overwhelms You.* New York: Carol Publishing Group, 1996.

Arora, R. C., et al. "Paroxetine Binding in the Blood Platelets of Post-traumatic Stress Disorder Patients." *Life Sciences* 53 (1993): 919–28.

"Asthma Linked to Post-traumatic Stress Disorder." ScienceDaily.com. www .sciencedaily.com/releases/2007/11/071115091713.htm. Accessed June 29, 2011.

Axe, Eleanor K., et al. "Major Depressive Disorder in Chronic Fatigue Syndrome: A CDC Surveillance Study." *Journal of Chronic Fatigue Syndrome* 12, no. 3 (2005): 7–23.

Bachner-Melman, Rachel, et al. "*AVPR1a* and *SLC64A* Gene Polymorphisms Are Associated with Creative Dance Performance." *PloS Genetics* 1, no. 3 (2005): e42.doi:10.1371/journal.pgen.0010042.

Barber, T. X. "Changing 'Unchangeable' Bodily Processes by Hypnotic Suggestions: A New Look at Hypnosis, Imaging and the Mind/Body Problem." *Advances* 1, no. 2 (1984): 7.

———. *Hypnosis: A Scientific Approach.* New York: Van Nostrand Reinhold, 1969.

Begley, Sharon. "The Depressing News about Antidepressants." *Newsweek*, February 8, 2010, sidebar, "The Placebo Effect," 40.

Bell, David S. "The Lyndonville Journal: Evaluating Blood Volume Studies—Some Thoughts." *Lyndonville News* (March 2000).

Benson, Herbert. *The Relaxation Response.* New York: William Morrow, 1975.

Benson H., J. B. Kotch, and K. D. Crassweller. "Relaxation Response: Bridge between Psychiatry and Medicine." *Medical Clinics of North America* 61 (1977): 929.

Berne, Katrina. *Chronic Fatigue Syndrome, Fibromyalgia, and Other Invisible Illnesses.* Salt Lake City, Utah: Hunter House, 2002.

Bernhardt, Peter, and Joel Isaacs. "The Bodymap: A Precise Diagnostic Tool for Psychotherapy." Bodynamic Institute USA. www.bodynamicusa.com/ documents/body_map.html. Accessed June 29, 2011.

Boivin, M. "Socioeconomic Impact of Irritable Bowel Syndrome in Canada." *Canadian Journal of Gastroenterology* 15 (October 2001): 8B–11B.

Boyles, Salynn. "CFC Linked to Childhood Trauma." WebMD, January 5, 2009. www.webmd.com/chronic-fatigue-syndrome/news/20090105/cfs-linked-to -childhood-trauma. Accessed June 29, 2011.

———. "Posttraumatic Stress, Fibromyalgia Linked." WebMD, June 10, 2004. www.webmd.com/fibromyalgia/news/20040610/posttraumatic-stress -fibromyalgia-linked. Accessed June 29, 2011.

"Brain Imaging Shows How Men and Women Cope Differently Under Stress." ScienceDaily.org, November 20, 2007. www.sciencedaily.com/releases/ 2007/11/071119170133.htm. Accessed June 29, 2011.

"Brain Response Differences in the Way Women with IBS Anticipate and

React to Pain." ScienceDaily.org, January 12, 2008. www.sciencedaily.com/releases/2008/01/080108183122.htm. Accessed June 29, 2011.

Brooke, Melody. "The Logic of Bodywork for Dissociation and Traumatic Stress." http://melodybrooke.com/docs/Logic%20of%20Bodywork.pdf. Accessed June 29, 2011.

Brooks J. S., and T. Scarano. "Transcendental Meditation in the Treatment of Post-Vietnam Adjustment." *Journal of Counseling and Development* 65 (1985): 212.

Broom, Brian. *Meaning*-Full *Disease*. London: Karnac Books, 2007.

———. *Somatic Illness and the Patient's Other Story*. New York: Free Association Books, 1997.

Brown, Harriet. "A Brain in the Head, and One in the Gut." *New York Times,* August 25, 2005. www.nytimes.com/2005/08/24/health/24iht-snbrain.html. Accessed June 29, 2011.

Bruce, Debra Fulghum. *Miracle Touch*. New York: Three Rivers Press, 2003.

Cahill, Larry. "His Brain, Her Brain." *Scientific American,* April 25, 2005, 40–47.

Carey, Bjorn. "Men and Women Really Do Think Differently." LiveScience, January 20, 2005. www.livescience.com/3808-men-women-differently.html. Accessed June 29, 2011.

Cardini, F., and H. Weixin. "Moxibustion for Correction of Breech Presentation: A Randomized Controlled Trial." *Journal of the American Medical Association* 280, no. 18 (1998): 1580–84.

Carroll, Roz. "Introduction and Background." Thinking through the Body. www.thinkbody.co.uk/intro.htm. Accessed June 29, 2011.

———. "Why Psychosomatization Is Complex: Going Beyond Cause-Effect." Thinking through the Body. www.thinkbody.co.uk/body-psych/psychosomatisation.htm. Accessed June 29, 2011.

Chaitow, Leon. "Chronic Fatigue/Fibromyalgia (Part 3): The Brain/Sleep Connection." Healthy.net. www.healthy.net/scr/article.asp?ID=589. Accessed June 29, 2011.

Chapman, C. Richard. "Pain, Suffering, and the Self." Fathom; Columbia University. www.fathom.com/feature/35587/index.html. Accessed June 29, 2011.

"Childhood Trauma and Chronic Fatigue Syndrome Risk Biologically Linked." ScienceDaily.org. www.sciencedaily.com/releases/2009/01/090105175025.htm. Accessed June 29, 2011.

"Chronic Fatigue Patients Show Lower Response to Placebos." ScienceDaily.org.

www.sciencedaily.com/releases/2005/04/050420090825.htm. Accessed June 29, 2011.

"Chronic Fatigue Syndrome Not Related to XMRV Retrovirus, Comprehensive Study Finds." ScienceDaily.org, May 4, 2011. www.sciencedaily.com/releases/2011/05/110504151337.htm. Accessed June 29, 2011.

Claire, Thomas. *Bodywork*. New York: William Morrow, 1995.

Cloninger, C. Robert. *Feeling Good: The Science of Well-Being*. New York: Oxford University Press, 2004.

Co, Stephen, and Eric B. Roberts, with John Merryman. *Your Hands Can Heal You*. New York: Free Press, 2002.

Cocke, Andrew. "Men and Women Remember Things in Different Ways." *Brain Work* (Charles A. Dana Foundation) (July–August 2002): 7.

Cole, J. Alexander, et al. "Migraine, Fibromyalgia, and Depression among People with IBS: A Prevalence Study." *BMC Gastroenterology* 6, no. 26 (September 28, 2006): doi:10.1186/1471-230X-6-26.

Connor, Kathryn M., and Marian L. Butterfield. "Post Traumatic Stress Disorder." *Focus* 1, no. 3 (2003): 247–62.

Cooper, M., and M. Aygen. "Effects of Meditation on Blood Cholesterol and Blood Pressure." *Journal of the Israel Medical Association* 95 (1978): 1.

Currey, Richard. "Research in the News: Ulcers—The Culprit Is *H. Pylori*." National Institutes of Health, Office of Science Education. http://science.education.nih.gov/home2.nsf/Educational+ResourcesResource+FormatsOnline+Resources+High+School/928BAB9A176A71B585256CCD00634489. Accessed June 29, 2011.

Damasio, Antonio R. *Descartes' Error: Emotion, Reason, and the Human Brain*. New York: G. P. Putnam's Sons, 1994.

Demitrack, Mark A., and Leslie J. Crofford. "Evidence for and Pathophysiological Implications of Hypothalamic-Pituitary-Adrenal Axis Dysregulation in Fibromyalgia and Chronic Fatigue Syndrome." *Annals of the New York Academy of Sciences* 840 (May 1998): 684–97.

DeNoon, Daniel J. "Childhood Trauma Raises CFS Risk." WebMD, November 6, 2006. www.webmd.com/content/article/129/117419.htm. Accessed June 29, 2011.

"Diagnosis: Do I Have CFS?" CFIDS Association of America. www.cfids.org/about-cfids/do-i-have-cfids.asp. Accessed June 29, 2011.

Diamond, John. *Life Energy*. New York: Dodd, Mead and Company, 1985.

"Diseases 101." American Academy of Allergy, Asthma and Immunology. www
.aaaai.org/patients/gallery/prevention.asp?item=1a. Accessed June 29, 2011.

"Doctors, Nurses Often Use Holistic Medicine for Themselves." MedicalXpress
.com. August 19, 2011. http://medicalxpress.com/news2011-08-doctors-nurses-
holistic-medicine.html. Accessed August 20, 2011.

Duff, Kat. *The Alchemy of Illness.* New York: Pantheon Books, 1993.

Durden-Smith, Jo, and Diane DeSimone. *Sex and the Brain.* New York: Arbor
House, 1983.

Dychtwald, Ken. *Bodymind.* Los Angeles: Jeremy P. Tarcher, 1977.

Eden, Donna, with David Feinstein. *Energy Medicine.* New York: Jeremy P. Tarcher/
Putnam, 1998.

Elias, Jason, and Katherine Ketcham. *The Five Elements of Self-Healing.* New York:
Harmony Books, 1998.

"Fibromyalgia Syndrome." *Health and Stress: The Monthly Newsletter of the American
Institute of Stress* 2 (1998): 2.

Field, Tiffany. *Touch.* Cambridge, Mass.: MIT Press, 2001.

Fitch, Pamela, and Trish Dryden. "Recovering Body and Soul from Post-traumatic
Stress Disorder." *Massage Therapy Journal* 39, no. 1 (2000): 41–62.

Fitzgerald, Michael, and Mark Bellgrove. "The Overlap between Alexithymia and
Asperger's Syndrome." *Journal of Autism and Developmental Disorders* 36, no.
4 (May 2006): 573–76.

Fogel, Alan. *The Psychophysiology of Self-Awareness.* New York and London:
W. W. Norton, 2009.

Ford, Clyde W. *Compassionate Touch: The Body's Role in Emotional Healing and
Recovery.* Berkeley, Calif.: North Atlantic Books, 1999.

Frattaroli, Elio. *Healing the Soul in the Age of the Brain.* New York: Viking Penguin,
2001.

"Further Doubt Cast on Virus Link to Chronic Fatigue." PhysOrg.com, February
16, 2010. www.physorg.com/news185552796.html. Accessed June 29, 2011.

Gao, Duo, ed. *Chinese Medicine.* New York: Thunder's Mouth Press, 1997.

Gardner, Amanda. "Genetics May Drive Chronic Fatigue Syndrome." HealingWell
.com. http://news.healingwell.com/index.php?p=news1&id=532266. Accessed
June 29, 2011.

"Gender Differences in Response to Pain." ScienceDaily.org, November 5, 2003.
www.sciencedaily.com/releases/2003/11/031105064626.htm. Accessed June
29, 2011.

Gershon, Michael. *The Second Brain: The Scientific Basis of Gut Instinct.* New York: HarperCollins, 1998.

Gilbert, Jonathan. "Breaking the Paradigm." *FM Frontiers* 13, no. 3 (2005).

Gonsalkorale, W. M., L. A. Houghton, and P. J. Whorwell. "Hypnotherapy in Irritable Bowel Syndrome: A Large-Scale Audit of a Clinical Service with Examination of Factors Influencing Responsiveness." *American Journal of Gastroenterology* 97 (2002): 954.

Gordon D. "The Fresh Face of Hypnosis: An Old Practice Finds New Uses." *Better Homes & Gardens,* February 2004.

Greco, C. M., T. E. Rudy, and S. Manzi. "Effects of a Stress-Reduction Program on Psychological Function, Pain, and Physical Function of Systemic Lupus Erythematosus Patients: A Randomized Controlled Trial." *Arthritis and Rheumatism* 51, no. 4 (2004): 625.

Green, Elmer, and Alyce Green. *Beyond Biofeedback.* New York: Delta, 1977.

Green, Elmer E., et al. "Anomalous Electrostatic Phenomena in Exceptional Subjects." *Subtle Energies* 2, no. 3 (1991): 69–94.

Greenspan, Miriam. *Healing through the Dark Emotions: The Wisdom of Grief, Faith, and Despair.* Boston: Shambhala, 2002.

Griffin, Susan. *What Her Body Thought: A Journey into the Shadows.* New York: HarperSanFrancisco, 1999.

Hadhazy, Adam. "Think Twice: How the Gut's 'Second Brain' Influences Mood and Well Being." Scientific American, February 21, 2010. www.scientificamerican .com/article.cfm?id=gut-second-brain. Accessed June 29, 2011.

Hajjar, I. J., M. Kotchen, and T. A. Kotchen. "Hypertension: Trends in Prevalence, Incidence and Control." *Annual Review of Public Health* 27 (2006): 465–90.

———. "Boundaries in the Mind: Implications for Mental and Physical Health." Grant proposal submitted to the Fetzer Institute, 1994.

———. *Boundaries in the Mind: A New Dimension of Personality.* New York: Basic Books, 1991.

Hartmann, Ernest. *Boundaries: A New Way to Look at the World.* Summerland, Calif.: CIRCC EverPress, 2011.

———. *Dreams and Nightmares: The New Theory of the Origin and Meaning of Dreams.* New York and London: Plenum Press, 1998.

Hartmann, Ernest, Robert Harrison, and Michael Zborowski. "Boundaries in the Mind: Past Research and Future Directions." *North American Journal of Psychology* 3 (June 2001): 347–68.

"Headaches and Fibromyalgia." Fibromyalgia-Symptoms.org. www.fibromyalgia -symptoms.org/fibromyalgia_chronic_headaches.html. Accessed June 29, 2011.

Heim, Christine, et al. "Pituitary-Adrenal and Autonomic Responses to Stress in Women After Sexual and Physical Abuse in Childhood." *Journal of the American Medical Association* 284 (2000): 592–97.

"*Helicobacter pylori* and Peptic Ulcer Disease: The Key to Cure." Centers for Disease Control and Prevention, Division of Bacterial Diseases. www.cdc.gov/ulcer/keytocure.htm. Accessed June 29, 2011.

Heller, Sharon. *Too Loud, Too Bright, Too Fast, Too Tight: What to Do If You Are Sensory Defensive in an Overstimulating World.* New York: HarperCollins, 2002.

Hill, Elisabeth, Sylvie Berthoz, and Uta Frith. "Brief Report: Cognitive Processing of Own Emotions in Individuals with Autistic Spectrum Disorder and in Their Relatives." *Journal of Autism and Developmental Disorders* 34, no. 2 (April 2004): 229–35.

Hillman, James. "A Psyche the Size of the Earth: A Psychological Foreword." In *Ecopsychology: Restoring the Earth, Healing the Mind,* edited by Theodore Roszak, Mary E. Gomes, and Allan D. Kanner. San Francisco: Sierra Club Books, 1995.

Hollifield, Michael, et al. "Acupuncture for Posttraumatic Stress Disorder: A Randomized Controlled Pilot Trial." *Journal of Nervous and Mental Disease* 195, no. 6 (June 2007): 504–13.

Hover-Kramer, Dorothea. *Creative Energies.* New York: W. W. Norton, 2002.

Humphrey, Nicholas. *A History of the Mind: Evolution and the Birth of Consciousness.* New York: Simon and Schuster, 1992.

"Hypnotherapy 'Can Help' Irritable Bowel Syndrome." BBC News. March 18, 2010. http://news.bbc.co.uk/2/hi/health/8572818.stm. Accessed August 17, 2011.

"Hypnotherapy Works for Bowel Pain." BBC News. October 22, 2003. http://news .bbc.co.uk/2/hi/health/3207972.stm. Accessed August 17, 2011.

"Irritable Bowel Syndrome." National Digestive Diseases Information Clearinghouse. http://digestive.niddk.nih.gov/ddiseases/pubs/ibs/. Accessed June 29, 2011.

"Irritable Bowel Syndrome's Possible Genetic Link Studied." ScienceDaily. www.sciencedaily.com/releases/2003/12/031211080446.htm. Accessed June 29, 2011.

"Is the Inability to Express Emotions Hereditary?" ScienceDaily.org. www .sciencedaily.com/releases/2007/11/071117114401.htm. Accessed June 29, 2011.

Ives, John A., and Wayne B. Jonas. "Energy and Medicine." In *Energy Medicine East and West: A Natural History of Qi,* edited by Marc S. Micozzi and David S. Mayor, 161–74. New York: Churchill Livingstone Elsevier, 2011.

Jawer, Michael A., with Marc S. Micozzi. *The Spiritual Anatomy of Emotion.* Rochester, Vt.: Park Street Press, 2009.

Johnson, Don Hanlon. "The Primacy of Experiential Practices in Body-Psychotherapy." www.donhanlonjohnson.com/articles/theprimacy.html. Accessed June 29, 2011.

Jones, Michael P., et al. "Alexithymia and Somatosensory Amplification in Functional Dyspepsia." *Psychosomatics* 45 (December 2004): 508–16.

Jordan, C. S., and K. T. Lenington. "Psychological Correlates of Eidetic Imagery and Induced Anxiety." *Journal of Mental Imagery* 3 (1979): 31.

Juhan, Deane. *Job's Body: A Handbook for Bodywork.* Barrytown, N.Y.: Barrytown/Station Hill Press, 2003.

Juhl, John H. "Fibromyalgia and the Serotonin Pathway." *Alternative Medicine Review* 3, no. 5 (1998): 367–75.

Jula, Antti, Jouko K. Salminen, and Simo Saarijärvi. "Alexithymia: A Facet of Essential Hypertension." *Hypertension* 33 (1999): 1057–61.

Jung, C. G. *An Answer to Job.* Princeton, New Jersey: Princeton University Press, 1973.

Kabat-Zinn, J. "Meditation." In Flowers, B. S., D. Grubin, and E. Meryman-Bruner, eds. *Healing and the Mind.* New York: Bantam/Doubleday, 1993.

———. "Mindfulness Meditation." In Goleman, Daniel and Joel Gurin, eds. *Mind-Body Medicine.* New York: Consumer Reports Books, 1993.

Kabat-Zinn, J., et al. "Four-Year Follow-Up of a Meditation-Based Program for the Self-Regulation of Chronic Pain." *Journal of Behavioral Medicine* 8 (1986): 163.

Kagan, Jerome, and Nancy Snidman. *The Long Shadow of Temperament.* Cambridge, Mass.: Belknap Press, 2004.

Kansky, Gail. "New Treatment for NMH." National CFIDS Foundation. www.ncf-net.org/forum/volumefall.htm. Accessed June 29, 2011.

Kaplan, K. H., et al. "The Impact of a Meditation-Based Stress Reduction Program on Fibromyalgia." *General Hospital Psychiatry* 15, no. 5 (1993): 284.

Kaplan, Norman M. "The Prevalence and Control of Hypertension." UpToDate. www.uptodate.com/patients/content/topic.do?topicKey=~IRUUUCmso2srZAg. Accessed June 29, 2011.

Kaptchuk, Ted J. *The Web That Has No Weaver: Understanding Chinese Medicine.* New York: Congdon and Weed, 1983.

Kaufmann, Walter, trans., ed. *The Portable Nietzsche*. New York: Viking Press, 1954.

Kessler, R. C., et al. "Posttraumatic Stress Disorder in the National Comorbidity Survey." *Archives of General Psychiatry* 52, no. 12 (December 1995): 1048–60.

Kidson, Ruth Lever. *Is Acupuncture Right for You?* Rochester, Vt.: Healing Arts Press, 2008.

Kline, Neil A., and Jeffrey Rausch. "Olfactory Precipitants of Flashback in Posttraumatic Stress Disorder: Case Reports." *Journal of Clinical Psychiatry* 67, no. 9 (September 1985): 383–84.

Koponen, Salla, et al. "Alexithymia after Traumatic Brain Injury: Its Relation to Magnetic Imagery Findings and Psychiatric Disorders." *Psychosomatic Medicine* 67, no. 5 (2005): 807–12.

Kosturek, Anna, et al. "Alexithymia and Somatic Amplification in Chronic Pain." *Psychosomatics* 39 (October 1998): 399–404.

Krieger, Dolores. *Therapeutic Touch as Transpersonal Healing*. New York: Lantern Books, 2002.

Kundera, Milan. *Immortality*. New York: Perennial Classics, 1999.

Kurcinka, Mary Sheedy. *Raising Your Spirited Child*. 2nd ed. New York: Harper, 2006.

Lance, James W. *Migraines and Other Headaches*. East Roseville, New South Wales, Australia: Simon and Schuster, 1998.

Lehrer, P. M., et al. "Biofeedback Treatment in Asthma." *Chest* 126, no. 2 (2004): 352.

Leskowitz, Eric. "Energy Medicine Perspectives on Phantom Pain." *Alternative and Complementary Therapies* 15, no. 2 (April 2009): 59–63.

———. "Phantom Pain: Subtle Energy Perspectives." *Subtle Energies and Energy Medicine* 8, no. 2 (2001): 125–52.

Lewandowski, W. A. "Patterning of Pain and Power with Guided Imagery." *Nursing Science Quarterly* 17, no. 3 (2004): 233.

"'Life Force' Linked to Body's Ability to Withstand Stress." University of Rochester Medical Center, June 17, 2009. www.urmc.rochester.edu/news/story/index .cfm?id=2522. Accessed June 29, 2011.

Lloyd, Robin. "Emotional Wiring Different in Men and Women." LiveScience. www.livescience.com/4085-emotional-wiring-men-women.html. Accessed June 29, 2011.

Lovejoy, C. Owen. "Models of Human Evolution." *Science* 217 (1982): 304–6.

Luria, A. R. *The Mind of a Mnemonist*. New York: Basic Books, 1968.

Lynch, James J. *The Language of the Heart: The Body's Response to Human Dialogue*. New York: Basic Books, 1985.

MacClaren, Kym. "Emotional Disorder and the Mind-Body Problem: A Case Study of Alexithymia." *Chiasmi International: Trilingual Studies Concerning Merleau-Ponty's Thought* 8 (2007): 139–55.

Mahoney, Michael. "Irritable Bowel Syndrome and Hypnotherapy." HealingWell.com. www.healingwell.com/library/ibs/mahoney1.asp. Accessed June 29, 2011.

Mann, Felix. *Acupuncture*. New York: Random House, 1971.

Martin, Paul. *The Healing Mind*. New York: St. Martin's Press, 1997.

Mason, A. A., and S. Black. "Allergic Skin Responses Abolished Under Treatment of Asthma and Hay Fever by Hypnosis." *Lancet* 1 (1958): 877.

Maté, Gabor. *When the Body Says No: Understanding the Stress-Disease Connection*. Hoboken, N.J.: John Wiley and Sons, 2003.

Maugh, Thomas H. "Chronic Fatigue Is in the Genes, Study Finds." *Los Angeles Times*, April 21, 2006, A1.

"Mayo Clinic Researchers Find Link between Irritable Bowel Syndrome (IBS), Alcoholism and Mental Illness." ScienceDaily. www.sciencedaily.com/releases/2004/11/041108020023.htm. Accessed June 29, 2011.

Mayor, David S., and Marc S. Micozzi, ed. *Energy Medicine East and West: A Natural History of Qi*. New York: Churchill Livingstone Elsevier, 2011.

McCown, Donald, and Marc S. Micozzi. *Everyday Mindfulness: A Practical Guide to Living in the Now*. Rochester, Vt.: Inner Traditions, 2012.

McCown, Donald, Dianne Reibel, and Marc S. Micozzi. *Teaching Mindfulness: A Practical Guide for Clinicians and Educators*. New York: Springer, 2010.

McCrae, Robert R., and Paul T. Costa, Jr. "Conceptions and Correlates of Openness to Experience." In *Handbook of Personality Psychology*, Hogan, R., J. A. Johnson, and S. R. Briggs, eds., 825–47. Orlando, Fl.: Academic Press, 1997.

McDougall, Joyce. *Theaters of the Mind: Truth and Illusion on the Psychoanalytic Stage*. New York: Brunner/Mazel, 1991.

———. *Theaters of the Body: A Psychoanalytic Approach to Psychosomatic Illness*. New York: Norton, 1989.

McManamy, John. "Depression in Women." McMan's Depression and Biopolar Web. www.mcmanweb.com/women_depression.html. Accessed June 29, 2011.

———. "FDA Antidepressant Suicide Warning." McMan's Depression and Biopolar Web. www.mcmanweb.com/FDA_suicide.htm. Accessed June 29, 2011.

Medow, Marvin. "Going with the Flow—Blood Flow, That Is." Webinar held by the CFIDS Association of America, with guest speaker Marvin Medow, Ph.D., March 25, 2010. Available at www.cfids.org/webinar/series2010.asp.

Melzack, Ronald. "Phantom Limbs." *Scientific American* (September 1997): 84–91.

———. "Phantom Limbs." *Scientific American* 266, no. 4 (April 1992): 120–26.

Meuret, A. E., et al. " Do Unexpected Panic Attacks Occur Spontaneously?" *Biological Psychiatry* (July 2011).

Micozzi, Marc S. *Celestial Healing: Energy, Mind and Spirit in Traditional Medicines of China, East and Southeast Asia.* London and Philadelphia: Singing Dragon Press, 2011.

———, ed. *Fundamentals of Complementary and Alternative Medicine.* 4th ed. St. Louis and Philadelphia: Elsevier-Saunders, 2011.

———. *Vital Healing: Energy, Mind and Spirit in Traditional Medicines of India, Tibet and the Middle East.* London and Philadelphia: Singing Dragon Press, 2011.

"Migraine and Fibromyalgia May Affect Nearly One-Quarter of Female Migraineurs." World Headache Alliance, March 28, 2006. www.w-h-a.org/index.cfm/spKey/archive/spId/C1F82490-0DF4-BDB7-774AFAD0CA635C0B.html. Accessed June 29, 2011.

"Migraine Headache Overview, Types of Migraine." Healthcommunities.com. www.healthcommunities.com/migraine/overview-of-migraine-headache.shtml. Accessed June 29, 2011.

"Migraine Headaches: Ways to Deal with the Pain." FamilyDoctor.org. http://familydoctor.org/online/famdocen/home/common/brain/disorders/127.html. Accessed June 29, 2011.

"Migrane Prevention and Treatment More Effective Than Most Realize." *Facts of Life* (newsletter) 7, no. 1 (2002).

Miller, R. "Nurses at Community Hospital Welcome Guided Imagery." *Dimensions in Critical Care Nursing* 22, no. 5 (2003): 225.

Montagu, Ashley. *Touching: The Human Significance of the Skin.* 2nd ed. New York: Harper and Row, 1978 (3rd ed. New York: Perennial Library, 1986).

Morris, Desmond. *The Human Zoo.* New York: McGraw-Hill, 1969.

Mueller, H. H., et al. "Treatment of Fibromyalgia Incorporating EEG-Driven Stimulation: A Clinical Outcomes Study." *Journal of Clinical Psychology* 57, no. 7 (2001): 933.

Muller, René. "When a Patient Has No Story to Tell: Alexithymia." *Psychiatric Times* 17, no. 7 (July 2000): 71–72.

Nahin, Richard L., et al. *Costs of Complementary and Alternative Medicine (CAM) and Frequency of Visits to CAM Practitioners: United States, 2007.* National Health Statistics Reports, No. 18. Hyattsville, Md.: National Center for Health Statistics, 2009. Available at www.cdc.gov/NCHS/data/nhsr/nhsr018.pdf. Accessed June 29, 2011.

Nathanielsz, Peter W. *Life in the Womb: Origin of Health and Disease.* Ithaca, N.Y.: Promethean, 1999.

"National Survey Sharpens Picture of Major Depression among U.S. Adults." ScienceDaily. www.sciencedaily.com/releases/2005/10/051004084117.htm. Accessed June 29, 2011.

Neri, I., et al., "Acupuncture Plus Moxibustion to Resolve Breech Presentation: A Randomized Controlled Study." Journal of Maternal-Fetal and Neonatal Medicine 15, no. 4 (2004): 247–52.

"New Hypothesis Proposed for Cause of Chronic Fatigue Syndrome." Ohio State University, Research News, October 28, 1998. http://researchnews.osu.edu/archive/cfs.htm. Accessed June 29, 2011.

"New Virus Is Not Linked to Chronic Fatigue Syndrome." PhysOrg.com, January 6, 2010. www.physorg.com/news181981582.html. Accessed June 29, 2011.

Nicolodi, M., and F. Sicuteri. "Fibromyalgia and Migraine, Two Faces of the Same Mechanism: Serotonin as the Common Clue for Pathogenesis and Therapy." *Advances in Experimental Medicine and Biology* 398 (1996): 373–79.

Norton, C., et al. "Randomized Controlled Trial of Biofeedback for Fecal Incontinence." *Gastroenterology* 125, no. 5 (2003): 1320.

O'Connor, Richard. *Undoing Perpetual Stress.* New York: Berkley Books, 2005.

Olness, K., and G. G. Gardner. *Hypnosis and Hypnotherapy with Children.* 2nd ed. Philadelphia: Saunders, 1988.

"One Gene Variant Puts Stressed Women at Risk for Depression; Has Opposite Effect in Men." ScienceDaily.org. www.sciencedaily.com/releases/2007/11/071129153320.htm. Accessed June 29, 2011.

Oschman, James L. *Energy Medicine: The Scientific Basis.* Edinburgh, U.K.: Churchill Livingstone, 2000.

"Overly Anxious and Driven People Prone to Irritable Bowel Syndrome." ScienceDaily.org. www.sciencedaily.com/releases/2007/02/070226095220.htm. Accessed June 29, 2011.

Oz, Mehmet, with Ron Arias and Lisa Oz. *Healing from the Heart.* New York: Dutton, 1998.

Paddock, Catharine. "Retrovirus Linked to Chronic Fatigue Syndrome." Medical News Today, October 9, 2009. www.medicalnewstoday.com/articles/166838 .php. Accessed June 29, 2011.

Palsson, Olafur. "Overview of Published Research to Date on Hypnosis for IBS." IBShypnosis.com. www.ibshypnosis.com/IBSresearch.html. Accessed June 29, 2011.

Parker, A. J., S. Wessely, and A. J. Cleare. "The Neuroendocrinology of Chronic Fatigue Syndrome and Fibromyalgia." Psychological Medicine 31, no. 8 (November 2001): 1331–45.

Paul, Annie Murphy. Origins: How the Nine Months before Birth Shape the Rest of Our Lives. New York: Free Press, 2010.

Pearce, Joseph Chilton. Evolution's End: Claiming the Potential of Our Intelligence. New York: HarperSanFrancisco, 1992.

Pearsall, Paul. The Heart's Code: Tapping the Wisdom and Power of Our Heart Energy. New York: Broadway Books, 1998.

Pearson, Helen. "Chronic Fatigue Has Genetic Roots." Nature News, April 21, 2006. BioEd Online, Baylor College of Medicine, www.bioedonline .org/news/news.cfm?art=2487. Accessed June 29, 2011.

Pelletier, Kenneth. The Best Alternative Medicine: What Works? What Does Not? New York: Simon and Schuster, 2000.

Pennebaker, James W. Opening Up: The Healing Power of Expressing Emotions. New York: Guilford Press, 1997.

Pert, Candace B. Molecules of Emotion: Why You Feel the Way You Feel. New York: Scribner, 1997.

Pfeffer, Cynthia R., et al. "Salivary Cortisol and Psychopathology in Children Bereaved by the September 11, 2001 Terror Attacks." Biological Psychiatry 61, no. 8 (April 15, 2007): 957–65.

"Post Traumatic Stress Disorder Fact Sheet." Sidran Institute. www.sidran.org/sub .cfm?contentID=66&sectionid=4. Accessed June 29, 2011.

"Prevalence." National Fibromyalgia Association. http://www.fmaware.org/site/ PageServera6cc.html?pagename=fibromyalgia_affected. Accessed August 17, 2011.

Ramasubbu, Rajamannar. "The Amnesia Gene." Scientific American, December 9, 2008. www.scientificamerican.com/article.cfm?id=the-amnesia-gene. Accessed June 29, 2011.

Reeves, Paula. Women's Intuition: Unlocking the Wisdom of the Body. Berkeley, Calif.: Conari, 1999.

Robotham, Julie. "Brain Link to Fatigue Syndrome," SMH.com.au, The Sydney Morning Herald. April 5, 2002. www.smh.com.au/articles/2002/05/03/1019441434909.html. Accessed June 29, 2011.

Rosch, Paul. "Some Psychological Perspectives on Traits, Temperament and Personality." *Health and Stress: The Monthly Newsletter of the American Institute of Stress* 8 (2001).

Roszak, Theodore, Mary E. Gomes, and Allan D. Kanner, eds. *Ecopsychology: Restoring the Earth, Healing the Mind.* San Francisco: Sierra Club Books, 1995.

Roth, Melissa J. "Irritable Bowel Syndrome and Hypnosis." HealingWell. www.healingwell.com/library/ibs/article.asp?author=roth&id=1. Accessed June 29, 2011.

Rothschild, Babette. *The Body Remembers.* New York: W. W. Norton, 2000.

Rubenfeld, Ilana. *The Listening Hand.* New York: Bantam Books, 2000.

Russell, I. J., et al. "Cerebrospinal Fluid Biogenic Amine Metabolites in Fibromyalgia/Fibrositis Syndrome and Rheumatoid Arthritis." *Arthritis Rheumatology* 35, no. 5 (May 1992): 550–56.

Sacks, Oliver. *Migraine.* Berkeley, Calif: University of California Press, 1992.

Scaer, Robert. "Observations on Traumatic Stress Utilizing the Model of the 'Whiplash Syndrome.'" *Bridges* 8, no. 1 (Spring 1997): 5–11. Available at Trauma Soma, http://traumasoma.com/excerpts/Observations%20on%20 Traumatic%20Stress.pdf. Accessed June 29, 2011.

Schirber, Michael. "Women Suffer More Than Men." LiveScience, July 6, 2005. www.livescience.com/3898-women-suffer-men.html. Accessed June 29, 2011.

Schneider, Antonius, et al. "Perception of Bodily Sensation as a Predictor of Treatment Response to Acupuncture for Postoperative Nausea and Vomiting Prophylaxis." *Journal of Alternative and Complementary Medicine* 11, no. 1 (February 2005), 119–25.

Schneider, R. H., et al. "A Randomized Controlled Trial of Stress Reduction for Hypertension in Older African Americans." *Hypertension* 26, no. 5 (1995): 820.

Schulz, Mona Lisa. *Awakening Intuition: Using Your Mind-Body Network for Insight and Healing.* New York: Harmony Books, 1998.

"Science of the Heart: Exploring the Role of the Heart in Human Performance." Institute of HeartMath. www.heartmath.org/research/science-of-the-heart/head-heart-interactions.html. Accessed June 29, 2011.

See, Emily. "New Evidence That Genetics Are Responsible for Chronic Fatigue Syndrome." *ProHealth*, May 2, 2006. www.prohealth.com/library/showarticle .cfm?id=7142&t=CFIDS_FM. Accessed June 29, 2011.

Selye, Hans. *The Stress of Life.* New York: McGraw-Hill, 1976.

Serrano, J., et al. "Alexithymia: A Relevant Psychological Variable in Near-Fatal Asthma." *European Respiratory Journal* 28 (2006): 296–302.

Servan-Schreiber, David. *The Instinct to Heal.* New York: Rodale, 2004.

"The Seven Developmental Stages." Bodynamic Institute USA. www.bodynamicusa .com/documents/41.html. Accessed June 29, 2011.

Sewall, Laura. "The Skill of Ecological Perception." In *Ecopsychology: Restoring the Earth, Healing the Mind,* edited by Theodore Roszak, Mary E. Gomes, and Allan D. Kanner, 201–15. San Francisco: Sierra Club Books, 1995.

"Sex Differences in the Brain's Serotonin System." ScienceDaily. www.sciencedaily .com/releases/2008/02/080213111043.htm. Accessed June 29, 2011.

Sharpe, M., et al. "Increased Brain Serotonin Function in Men with Chronic Fatigue Syndrome." *British Medical Journal* 315 (1997): 164–65.

Sharples, Tiffany. "Wish Fulfillment? No. But Dreams Do Have Meaning." Time, June 15, 2009. www.time.com/time/health/article/0,8599,1904561,00.html. Accessed June 29, 2011.

Sheikh, Anees A. *Imagery: Current Theory, Research and Application.* New York: John Wiley and Sons, 1983.

Shin, Lisa M., et al. "Regional Cerebral Blood Flow During Script-Driven Imagery in Childhood Sexual Abuse-Related PTSD: A PET Investigation." *American Journal of Psychiatry* 156 (April 1999): 575–84.

Sifneos, Peter E. "The Prevalence of 'Alexithymic' Characteristics in Psychosomatic Patients." *Psychotherapy and Psychosomatics* 22 (1973): 255–62.

Silverman, Marnie N., et al. "Neuroendocrine and Immune Contributors to Fatigue." *PM & R: The Journal of Injury, Function, and Rehabilitation* 2, no. 5 (May 2010): 338–46.

Solomon, George Freeman. "Psychoneuroimmunology and Chronic Fatigue Syndrome: Toward New Models of Disease." *Journal of Chronic Fatigue Syndrome* 1, no. 1 (1995): 7.

Sperber, A. D., et al. "Fibromyalgia in the Irritable Bowel Syndrome: Studies of Prevalence and Clinical Implications." *American Journal of Gastroenterology* 94 (1999): 3541–46.

Stewart, Walter F., et al. "Prevalence of Migraine Headache in the United States." *Journal of the American Medical Association* 267, no. 1 (January 1, 1992): 64–69.

Streeten, David H. P., and David S. Bell. "Circulating Blood Volume in Chronic Fatigue Syndrome." *Journal of Chronic Fatigue Syndrome* 4, no. 1 (1998): 3–11.

Swaminathan, Nikhil. "A Gene to Better Remember Traumatic Events." Scientific American, July 30, 2007. www.scientificamerican.com/article.cfm?id=gene-to-remember-traumatic-events. Accessed June 29, 2011.

Tepper, Stewart J. "Migraine Prevalence and Disease Burden." JournalWatch Specialties. http://neurology.jwatch.org/cgi/content/full/2007/410/3. Accessed June 29, 2011.

Tietjen, Gretchen, et al. "Childhood Maltreatment and Migraine (Part II): Emotional Abuse as a Risk Factor for Headache Chronification." Headache 50, no. 1 (January 2010): 32–41.

Todarello, Orlando, et al. "Alexithymia in Essential Hypertensive and Psychiatric Outpatients: A Comparative Study." Journal of Psychosomatic Research 39, no. 8 (November 1995): 987–94.

Toffler, Alvin. Future Shock. New York: Random House, 1970.

Topf, Linda Noble, with Hal Zina Bennett. You Are Not Your Illness. New York: Simon and Schuster, 1995.

Twain, Mark. Following the Equator: A Journey Around the World. New York: Dover, 1989.

"Understanding Migraines." Excedrin.com. www.excedrin.com/headache_center/migraines_understanding.shtml. Accessed June 29, 2011.

Van de Putte, Elise M., et al. "Alexithymia in Adolescents with Chronic Fatigue Syndrome." Journal of Psychosomatic Research 63, no. 4 (October 2007): 377–80.

Van Den Eede, Filip, et al. "Hypothalamic-Pituitary-Adrenal Axis Function in Chronic Fatigue Syndrome." Neuropsychobiology 55, no. 2 (June 2007): 112–20.

Van Houdenhove, Boudewijn, et al. "Victimization in Chronic Fatigue Syndrome and Fibromyalgia in Tertiary Care." Psychosomatics 42 (February 2001): 21–28.

Vance, Erik. "Seeking to Illuminate the Mysterious Placebo Effect." New York Times, June 21, 2010. www.nytimes.com/2010/06/22/health/22prof.html?_r=1.

Vas, J., et al., "Correction of Nonvertex Presentation with Moxibustion: A Systematic Review and Metaanalysis." American Journal of Obstetrics and Gynecology 201, no. 3 (2009): 241–59.

Velle, Weiert. "Sex Differences in Sensory Functions." Perspectives in Biology and Medicine 30, no. 4 (1987): 490–522.

Vernon, Suzanne D. "Association-Funded Researchers Making Headway." CFIDS Association of America. http://cfids.org/cfidslink/2010/010605.asp. Accessed June 29, 2011.

Wallace, Daniel J., and Janice Brock Wallace. *All about Fibromyalgia*. New York: Oxford University Press, 2002.

Watkins, Alan D. "The Electrical Heart: Energy in Cardiac Health and Disease." In *Energy Medicine East and West: A Natural History of Qi,* edited by Marc S. Micozzi and David S. Mayor, 305–18. New York: Churchill Livingstone Elsevier, 2011.

Weissbecker, Inka, et al. "Childhood Trauma and Dirurnal Cortisol Disruption in Fibromyalgia Syndrome." *Psychoneuroendocrinology* 31, no. 3 (2006): 312–24.

Whalley, Matthew. "Measurement of Hypnosis and Hypnotisability." Hypnosis and Suggestion. www.hypnosisandsuggestion.org/measurement.html. Accessed June 29, 2011.

White, K. D. "Salivation: the Significance of Imagery in its Voluntary Control." *Psychophysiology* 15, no. 3 (1978): 196.

Whorwell, Peter J. "Hypnotherapy for Functional Gastrointestinal Disorders." HypnoGenesis. www.hypnos.co.uk/hypnomag/whorwell.htm. Accessed June 29, 2011.

Wilson, Sheryl C., and Theodore X. Barber. "The Fantasy-Prone Personality: Implications for Understanding Imagery, Hypnosis, and Parapsychological Phenomena." In *Imagery: Current Theory, Research and Application,* edited by Anees A. Sheikh, 340–87. New York: John Wiley and Sons, 1983.

Wolfe, F., et al. "Serotonin Levels, Pain Threshold, and Fibromyalgia Symptoms in the General Population." *Journal of Rheumatology* 24, no. 3 (March 1997): 555–59.

"Women More Depressed and Men More Impulsive with Reduced Serotonin Functioning," ScienceDaily.org. www.sciencedaily.com/releases/2007/09/070917112504.htm. Accessed June 29, 2011.

Yehuda, Rachel. "Psychoneuroendocrinology of Post-Traumatic Stress Disorder." *The Psychiatric Clinics of North America* 21 (1998): 359–79.

Yunus, Mohammad. "Are Fibromyalgia and Other Chronic Conditions Associated?" ProHealth. June 8, 2000. www.prohealth.com/fibromyalgia/library/showarticle.cfm?id=1406&t=CFIDS_FM. Accessed June 29, 2011.

INDEX

ABOUT THE AUTHORS

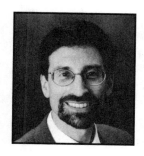

Michael A. Jawer is an emotion researcher. Since 1998 he has been delving in to the subject of how bodily feeling underlies consciousness and how the energy of feelings plays an integral role in immunity, stress reactions, and numerous psychosomatic conditions, including migraine headache, synesthesia (overlapping senses), chronic fatigue, phantom pain, and post-traumatic stress disorder.

A professional communicator, Jawer has written on diverse subjects for trade and professional associations as well as the federal government. He is an expert on "sick building syndrome" and has been researching connections with other forms of sensitivity. His book *The Spiritual Anatomy of Emotion* (coauthored with Marc Micozzi) supplies a bold and timely counter to neuroscience's assertion that the brain rules the body and alone determines the self.

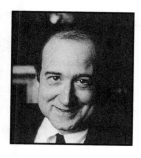

Marc Micozzi, M.D., Ph.D., a national leader in the emerging field of complementary, alternative, and integrative medicine (CAM), is a professor of physiology and biophysics at the Georgetown University School of Medicine and the medical editor and coauthor (with Michael Jawer) of *The Spiritual Anatomy of Emotion*. Dr. Micozzi was the founding editor in chief of the first U.S. journal on the subject of CAM in 1994, and he organized and edited the first U.S. textbook, *Fundamentals of Complementary & Alternative Medicine* (1996).

Prior to his work in CAM, Dr. Micozzi worked as a senior investigator in the Cancer Prevention Studies Branch of the National Cancer Institute from 1984–1986 and as director of the National Museum of Health and Medicine (affiliated with the National Institutes of Health). He also served as executive director of the Center for Integrative Medicine at Thomas Jefferson University Hospital and as executive director of the College of Physicians of Philadelphia.

Currently based in Washington, D.C., he now works to educate policymakers, health care professionals, and the general public about needs and opportunities for integrative medicine to benefit all Americans

Visit the authors on this book's website at **www.YourEmotionalType.com.**

BOOKS OF RELATED INTEREST

The Spiritual Anatomy of Emotion
How Feelings Link the Brain, the Body, and the Sixth Sense
by Michael A. Jawer with Marc S. Micozzi, M.D., Ph.D.

New World Mindfulness
From the Founding Fathers, Emerson, and Thoreau
to Your Personal Practice
by Donald McCown and Marc S. Micozzi, M.D., Ph.D.

Walking Your Blues Away
How to Heal the Mind and Create Emotional Well-Being
by Thom Hartmann

Breathing
Expanding Your Power and Energy
by Michael Sky

Is Acupuncture Right for You?
What It Is, Why It Works, and How It Can Help You
by Ruth Lever Kidson

Bioharmonic Self-Massage
How to Harmonize Your Mental, Emotional, and Physical Energies
by Yves Bligny

**Integrative Therapies for Fibromyalgia,
Chronic Fatigue Syndrome, and Myofascial Pain**
The Mind-Body Connection
by Celeste Cooper, R.N., and Jeffrey Miller, Ph.D.

Trigger Point Self-Care Manual
For Pain-Free Movement
by Donna Finando, L.Ac., L.M.T.

Inner Traditions • Bear & Company
P.O. Box 388
Rochester, VT 05767
1-800-246-8648
www.InnerTraditions.com

Or contact your local bookseller

Bodymind Maps

Both West and East have ways of charting the evolution of body-mind. While the charting systems are very different, they also have an overall similarity. Figure 2 reflects an Eastern perspective and figure 1 a predominantly Western view. We can see that the aim in both cases is to better understand—wholistically—the way our bodymind functions.

Figure 1 was produced by a school of body psychotherapists concerned with muscle tone in the clients they see. Figure 2 shows the principal acupuncture meridians and acupoints.

For a complete discussion of the content and use of these illustrations, see chapter 8, Pushing Boundaries, pages 104–5.

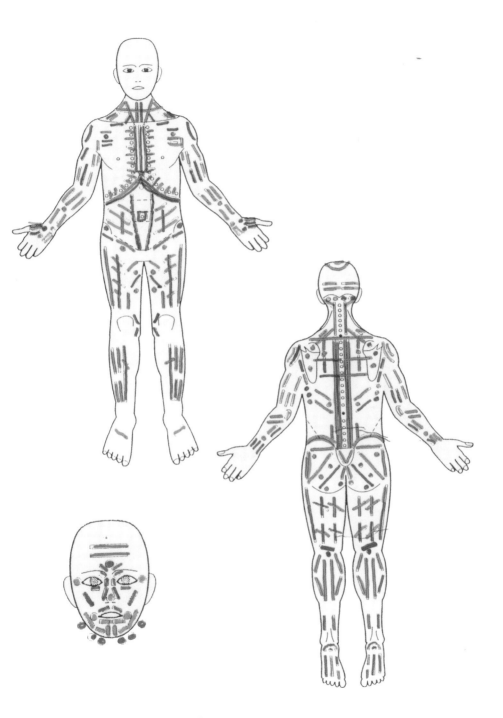

Figure 1. Bodymap of a Biodynamic client.
Image provided by Bodynamic Institute USA.

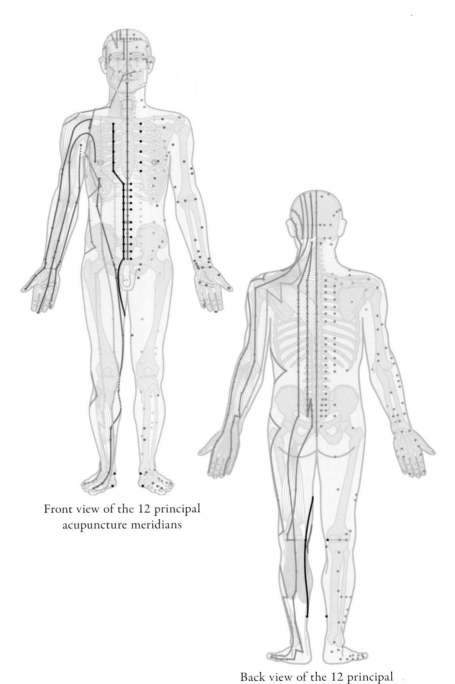

Front view of the 12 principal
acupuncture meridians

Back view of the 12 principal
acupuncture meridians

Figure 2. Chinese meridians